SURROUNDED
L*by*OVE

SURROUNDED
L*by*OVE

*One Family's Journey
Through Stroke Recovery*

Lori Martin Williams

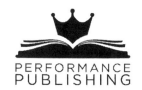

PERFORMANCE
PUBLISHING

To Mark, Chris and Abby

"For I know the plans I have for you," declares the Lord, "plans to prosper you and not to harm you, plans to give you hope and a future."
Jeremiah 29:11

Contents

Introduction

The year 2022 started off with a bang. I declared it my year of growth, both personally and professionally.

My senior placement business was booming and my podcast, *Aging in Style with Lori Williams*, was growing in popularity. I was moving my office to a larger space the first of January. My new lease was signed and I was excited about what the New Year would bring.

I had also made the decision to share the knowledge gained through my 17+ years of experience in senior living by writing a book to serve as a guide through the maze of senior housing and services. I envisioned it as sort of a map explaining the different types of housing and services available to older adults. I also planned to share common pitfalls they may encounter along the way, and how to avoid them. I was nervous and excited about the prospect of writing my first book.

I've always loved to write, and have secretly wanted to be an author since I was in second grade and wrote my highly acclaimed (by my teacher) short story, "I'm Riding my Bicycle to the Moon." No, I'm not going to share it here, but I would if I knew where it was!

After many years of thinking about writing a book, I finally felt clear on the topic and made the decision to do it. I even proudly announced publicly that I was on my way to publishing my first book and adding "Author" to my list of accomplishments.

Writing a book requires great discipline, and by October 2022, I had only written a handful of chapters. I was annoyed with myself, because I kept losing focus and instead of writing, I would find myself out shopping for shoes with my sister-in-law, or binging the latest Netflix show with my husband. I set a tough deadline for myself: finish the book by the end of the year.

Spoiler alert…I did NOT finish the book.

My life and the lives of my family were turned completely upside down on Christmas Day 2022, when my husband, Mark, had the first in a series of four strokes. No one believes that a catastrophic event will befall them or their loved ones – especially, when they are still relatively young. At the time of his strokes, Mark was only 62 and I was 58.

My family and I are now over a year into a journey we never expected to be on. Our lives have been completely and forever changed.

I've spent years listening to other people's stories and assisting them in finding help for their loved ones, and can say it's truly a humbling experience to be the one needing the help. I'm thankful that, due to my experience and an incredible network of friends who work in healthcare, finding resources has been a bit easier for me. However, it has made me keenly aware of how difficult this journey is for those who don't have the same connections and knowledge.

When a loved one is critically ill, you are under incredible stress, struggling to understand all of the medical jargon being thrown at you, plus having to make decisions about their care. Navigating your way through hospitals, rehabs, and then ultimately taking on the role of caregiver is a lot for anyone to deal with.

I tried several times to return to the book I was initially writing about senior living, but my mind would always end up focusing on others who were experiencing what my family and I were going through. As difficult as this journey has been for us, I have learned a lot that I felt could benefit others just beginning a similar unexpected and unwelcome journey.

I have a deep faith and belief in God, and honestly felt that He kept putting this on my heart. Finally, I stopped fighting it by trying to write the other book, and realized this is the book that needed to be written, and I was the one to write it.

In this book, I tell my family's story of catastrophic illness and the road to recovery. It's not an easy story to tell, but I hope it will serve two purposes – one, as a guide and encouragement for others going through similar situations and two, as a source of inspiration. I believe that there is always something positive to be found even in the most difficult of times.

This book is dedicated to my family, friends and neighbors, too many to list, who surrounded my family with love as the world we knew came crumbling down. There are no words to express our gratitude for the love, prayers, meals, fundraisers, etc., that were showered upon us through such a dark time. I want all of you to know that you were the light for us and kept us positive and moving forward when we were at our lowest.

CHAPTER 1

The Moment Life Changed

Christmas Day 2022
7:00 p.m.

The date and time are burned into my memory.

How many times have I relived that entire day, asking myself why did this happen and why, of all days, on Christmas Day? Wondering what signs I may have missed, or what I could have done differently. Wishing that time machines truly existed so I could hop in one and travel back to 6:59 p.m. when our family was still "us".

Christmas 2022 was very low-key for our family, and honestly it was probably a bit on the boring side. We had toyed with plans to join our extended family in Mississippi for the holidays, but we didn't want to leave our 11-month-old golden retriever puppy with a sitter. And the thought of driving ten hours with four of us in a car plus an 85-pound energetic pup appealed to none of us. Christmas morning the kids, 26-year-old Chris and 19-year-old Abby, slept in. I got up early and made a breakfast casserole (sausage, biscuits, and gravy) that I found on *Pinterest*. I figured we'd all fill up on a big breakfast and eat a late dinner. Mark and I watched a movie on Netflix – I have no memory of what it was.

However, I do remember how normal everything was as we sat in our regular TV viewing spots in our family room – Mark in his recliner and me on the couch, cozily wrapped in a warm blanket.

There was no feeling of impending doom.

At some point, I put a Honey Baked ham in the oven and got to work on a scalloped potato recipe Abby had found and asked me to make. As I recall, she was supposed to help me with it, but had gone MIA, sleeping no doubt, as most college students do when home on Christmas break.

I recruited Mark into helping me with the casserole, specifically peeling the potatoes and thinly slicing them with a mandoline. Not two minutes into this, Mark cut his hand. It wasn't terribly deep, but he did bleed, which earned him an immediate release from food prep. I finished up the casserole and placed it in the oven. If all had gone according to plan, dinner would've been ready by 6:00 – however, those darn scalloped potatoes were taking forever to cook.

While we were waiting on the potatoes, we called our extended family to wish them a Merry Christmas. I remember Mark going upstairs to his office to call his sister and niece.

Finally, dinner was ready! I remember how good it smelled and how hungry I was. I'd only had a slice of breakfast casserole and some fruit earlier in the morning. I had also popped about half a box of chocolate covered cherries in my mouth throughout the day…don't judge me, it was Christmas!

In our kitchen we have a long island where I had arranged all of the food and put the plates out buffet-style. We were all starving by this time, of course. Normally, we would plate our food, sit at the table and Mark would say the blessing. However, since we were eating so late I told everyone to stay where they were around the island and asked Mark to say the blessing.

This is the moment where life as we knew it came to an abrupt end.

I was standing on one side of the island, Mark was on the other, and I was facing him. Chris was on the same side as Mark and Abby was on my side. I remember glancing at the large clock hanging on the wall in our family room and noting that it was 7:00 p.m. I asked Mark to say the blessing. His mouth opened and closed a few times, and then he had a perplexed look on his face. The words he got out were, "You say it." I immediately felt a sense of alarm, and asked him to say something else. Whatever he said was slurred and unintelligible and I immediately knew what was happening. I remember telling him…

"You're having a stroke."

Years ago, there was a commercial about recognizing the signs of a stroke, for whatever reason I never forgot it. The acronym they used was FAST – which stands for Face (Is there drooping on one side?), Arms (Can both arms be lifted evenly?), Speech (Is it slurred?), and Time (Get help fast!).

The only sign that Mark had was slurred speech, but I knew without a doubt he was having a stroke. I looked at the kids who both were wide eyed with shocked looks on their precious faces. I asked them, "Are you hearing this?" They both silently nodded. I told Chris to stand next to Mark to support him in case he became weak, while I ran to put on my shoes and grab my purse and his wallet.

In retrospect, I should've had him sit down and called 911, but all that was going through my mind was get him to the hospital FAST. I remember he walked to the car, buckled his seat belt on his own and was completely silent. I was backing out of the driveway while simultaneously calling my friend Karyl, who works in hospice. She answered and I blurted out, "Mark's having a stroke, which hospital should I go to?" Without hesitation she told me the closest, so I headed to the hospital driving like a bat out of hell. I should mention that my family calls me a "grandma driver" due to my cautious and turtle-like pace of driving. No "grandma driving" that night – I got him to the hospital in under three minutes.

I drove to the Emergency Room entrance, outwardly remaining calm. Mark was still able to walk, as we entered the ER, I was surprised to see not one person in the waiting room. Before the receptionist at the front desk could say a word, I blurted out, "He's having a stroke!" She looked at me like I was the biggest idiot in the world and said in a patronizing tone, "And why do you think he's having a stroke?" At this point I was losing my calm as the seriousness of the situation was sinking in, so I yelled at her, "BECAUSE HE IS!" I must've been a bit louder than I intended and probably had a panicked tone, because immediately medical staff appeared and took Mark into a room where they began taking his vitals and asking questions. Within minutes I heard *CODE STROKE* over the loud speaker and doctors and nurses were rushing into the room. I relayed what had happened, as they began the stroke protocol…

Mr. Williams, can you smile? (checking to see if one side of his face was drooping).
Mr. Williams, can you raise both of your arms? (checking for weakness on one or both sides).
Mr. Williams, can you tell us your name and date of birth? (checking for difficulty with speech).

He could do all of these, except state his name or date of birth.

At this point, someone asked me if I had left my car at the entrance of the ER. Yep, I had pretty much abandoned it, the passenger door hanging wide open. They asked me to please move it, and as I drove to a parking space, I called my brother Craig to tell him what was going on. I was gone for just a few minutes, but when I walked back into the room I had left Mark in, he was gone. They had taken him for an MRI. After what felt like an eternity, a nurse came to get me and took me to another room in the ER where they had moved Mark.

The doctor was again asking him, "What is your name and your date of birth?" He had this look on his face of confusion because he couldn't answer either question, and then he would give a little laugh, kind of like he couldn't believe the absurdity of not being able to recall his own name or birth-date. Doctors and nurses were in and out – it's all kind of a blur – but I remember one of the doctors informing me that the hospital we were in did not have a neurology department and Mark had definitely had a stroke.

The doctor was on the phone communicating with a neurologist at their sister hospital thirty minutes away in Plano and they had determined it would be best to give him the clot busting drug TPA or Tenecteplase. I had heard of this drug and knew that if given within the first two hours it could save your life. However, in my naïveté, I thought if the drug is given, it would "stop" the stroke and everything will go back to normal. *Oh, If only it worked that way.*

I will share more information on strokes and the damage they do in a later chapter.

So, we now had a plan in place and Mark needed the clot-buster drug. However, at this point, he could not sign the paperwork and did not seem to understand what the doctor was explaining to him about his condition. The doctor turned to me and said, "You have to make the decision for him, and you need to know there are significant risks, but this is his best shot, and the benefits outweigh the risks."

I honestly never imagined that I would be in the position of making life or death decisions for my husband.

I asked the doctor about the risks and he stated that excessive bleeding is the biggest concern because the drug would thin his blood. We need to make sure he doesn't have a fall, and if he has cuts anywhere, they will begin to bleed. *Remember, he cut his hand earlier in the day while helping me prepare the scalloped potatoes?*

The drug was then administered through IV and I texted the kids and my brother Craig to let them know what was happening.

I remember standing in this small room in the ER, sort of plastered up against the wall since there were so many people coming in and out. At one point, I heard a nurse say CareFlite is twenty minutes out. *Wait...what?? They are transporting Mark by helicopter to another hospital? Okay, this is VERY serious.*

The helicopter arrived and the crew came in with the transfer gurney, I remember the pilot saying, "It's the size of an ironing board," and it was. My husband is a good-sized guy and I wondered how on earth they were going to fit him on such a tiny gurney. I told Mark I loved him and would meet him at the next hospital as they got him ready for transport. They took him out one set of doors to the helicopter as I was told to go out the opposite doors through the ER. I can't explain the feeling of shock, numbness and disbelief. Is this really happening? As I walked through the ER, the receptionist who had been so rude when we first arrived, called out that she was sorry and hoped he would be okay. I thanked her and said I hoped so too.

As I walked out to the parking lot, I could see them loading Mark into the helicopter. It was a freezing cold night, and by this time it was about 9:30. I called the kids to tell them that daddy had just been loaded into the helicopter and that I would stop at the house to get my coat before driving to the next hospital. I stood outside of my car and watched the helicopter take off with my husband in it, praying that he would be okay. *It was beyond surreal.*

Feeling completely numb, I drove to my house. I was so scared for Mark and so sad for my kids. I had an overwhelming need to hug them and make sure they were okay. I walked into the kitchen and they both looked so young and scared. Sweet

Abby had packed me a bag of essentials. I don't remember everything that was in it, but there was a blanket which came in very handy. We have no family locally, and I felt awful leaving them, especially Abby, who is very sensitive and the biggest "daddy's girl" ever. I called my neighbors Marco and Sole, as I drove to the hospital where Mark had been taken. They are like family and I knew they'd check on Chris and Abby and make sure they were okay. I found out later that Sole had rushed to our house immediately after I called with cookies and hugs for the kids.

I don't remember much of the drive to the hospital he was taken to, but I quickly located Mark in the ER. By this point the clot buster drug had done its thing and he was talking to me, which was amazing! He was also bleeding profusely out of the cut in his hand and some other minor cuts on his arm. That was pretty freaky to be honest. I remember the nurse had to bandage up his hand because it was bleeding so much. He was admitted into the Intensive Care Unit (ICU) and once he was settled into his room I was allowed to join him.

At this point he was still able to walk and had full use of his right side. The nurse told me that it was very important that he not fall because of the bleeding that would occur due to the clot-buster drug. I felt such relief because he looked so much better and he was talking with just a slight slur. He said to me, with this look of awe on his face, "That was so weird." The stroke itself wasn't painful, but everything had been so confusing for him.

Mark then told me that strange things had started prior to not being able to say the blessing at dinner. Turns out, when he had gone upstairs to his office to call his niece and sister he was trying to enter their numbers into his phone, but it wasn't making sense to him. Thank God I called him down to dinner when I did. I shudder to think what would've happened if he had been up there for hours and I'd had no clue that he was having a stroke.

We settled into the ICU, as settled as you can be in an ICU. Mark's room was the first one as you entered the unit. My most vivid memory is how loud it was – constant beeping of machines, doors clanging, the sound of equipment being rolled around – truly the most stressful environment I think I have ever been in. I sat in a chair all night covered in the blanket Abby had sent with me. Mark slept some, but of course the nurses were popping in the room constantly to check his vitals. I felt cold and wired, adrenaline I suppose as I tried to process what had happened over the past several hours. I felt a bit sick to my stomach too – a combination of stress and that my last meal had been half a box of chocolate covered cherries earlier in the day.

After what felt like an eternity, morning arrived. The neurologist, a very kind man that I will always remember, came in to discuss the results of Mark's tests. It was good news, all things considered. It was a small stroke, the clot-buster drug did what it was supposed to do. He would need some therapy to address the slight slur to his speech and some weakness on his right side, but by next Christmas it would be like it never happened. *Yes! Great news!* I breathed a huge sigh of relief.

I texted the latest update to my dear friend from college, Kathy Messenger. She's a neurologist in Mississippi and I had been texting her all night, relaying all of the medical jargon to her for interpretation. My sister-in-law Dianne is a Nurse Anesthetist and I was also sending her Mark's vitals and anything else the doctors or nurses told me. Everyone agreed, things were looking up and it seemed like Mark had dodged a bullet, and that he would have a good outcome!

By early afternoon, my neighbor Sole had arrived to sit with Mark so I could run home for a few hours to check on the kids and take a much needed shower.

I walked in the house and had a long group hug with the kids. Their worried sweet faces about broke my heart. They had cleaned up and put away all of the food from the forgotten Christmas dinner. I had zero appetite and knew there was no way I could eat one bite of that meal ever. I showered, took about a one hour nap and headed back to the hospital.

I will never forget that drive back, because I had such an incredible feeling of relief. This could've been really bad, but we caught it in time and he's okay. *Thank God!*

Back in ICU, I hugged Sole and thanked her for coming to sit with Mark. Once she left, Mark said he needed to go to the bathroom. There was a toilet in his room with a half curtain to pull around it. I was nervous about him getting up without a nurse present – thoughts of the clot-buster drug and the warnings of falling were at the forefront of my mind. He refused any help and became angry with me. I stood close by just in case he needed help. I breathed a sigh of relief when he returned safely to his chair. That relief was short-lived.

I was sitting directly across from Mark and we were talking. As I looked at him, I saw his entire right side suddenly droop – his mouth, his arm, his leg. I opened the door and yelled for a nurse and then ran to his side to make sure he wouldn't fall out of the chair. He tried to speak, but it was slurred and made no sense. His eyes were confused and scared.

All available medical staff converged into the room, as I made myself as small as possible in a corner. It was obvious that he'd had another stroke, and I knew this time it was very bad. What I didn't know until later was that he'd had a "stroke shower" which means he had three more strokes all at the same time. Four strokes total.

He was now paralyzed on his right side, the right side of his face twisted and drooping to the right and no longer coherent.

In an instant, we had gone from a minor stroke and the prognosis that "he will be back to normal by next Christmas"… to massive strokes and serious disability.

Mercifully, for him, he has no memory of any of this. *I wish I could say the same.*

CHAPTER 2

Our Family Story

Mark and I met in January 1988. I've always loved telling the story because it's definitely a meet cute! I'm from Baton Rouge, Louisiana, and Mark had moved there from the Fort Worth, Texas, area in 1987, to open an office for Transamerica (Real Estate Tax Service Division). I was finishing up my last year at LSU, working part time, and dating a guy my parents did not approve of.

I happened to stop by my parents' house to pick something up and found my mom preparing a feast. My mom is an incredible cook and I was a starving college student, so of course the smell of delicious food caught my attention. This wasn't just a regular dinner she was cooking, she had invited her boss and some other people from her office over for a dinner party. *Boring!* I figured her boss was some bald, 40-year-old dude…so, I was prepared to leave as quickly as possible to go meet the boyfriend no one approved of, yet I was still seeing on the downlow. (*Scandalous, I know!*)

The doorbell rang and my mom asked me to answer it for her. I opened the door and there stood this good-looking, dark-haired, young guy in his late 20's, wearing a blue sweatshirt and jeans. I immediately thought, *I'm going to marry this guy.* He said, "Hi, I'm Mark Williams." *Holy crap, this is my mom's boss??* Thankfully, my dad took over as I was pretty much just staring at Mark. I ran to the kitchen and said to my mom, "Why didn't you mention that your boss is young and cute? And I'm staying for dinner!" My mom just shook her head, but I successfully finagled an invitation and a seat right next to Mark at the dinner table. (Oh, and I stood up the boyfriend.) This was before cell phones and he wouldn't dare call my parents' house.

I'd like to say that Mark was just as enamored with me, but that was not the case. We had a nice conversation, and I thought he showed some interest, but he didn't ask me out. I couldn't stop thinking about him, so I suddenly began showing up at my mom's office. I'm not going to lie, I didn't have any idea where she worked prior to meeting her boss. One day in February, my mom was home and asked if I'd run up to her office to pick up her check (remember this was the '80's before direct deposit). I made sure my big 80's spiral-permed hair was sufficiently coated in Aqua Net, put on the cutest pale pink sweater dress with shoulder pads and my red wool coat, and headed up to her office. *Y'all, I was looking good!*

Mark had a secretary named Cecilia who was doing her best matchmaking on my behalf. She gave me a huge smile and told me to go into his office. I can still see him sitting behind his big desk looking so important. I confidently said, "Hi, I'm here to pick up my mom's check." His response, "Who's your mom?"

Oh my God. What? I couldn't respond, but I'm sure the look on my face was enough, because he started laughing and said, "I know who you are." This is the moment I learned that Mark Williams was a practical joker!

After that, I backed off on my efforts to get him to ask me out. I figured this guy is just not into me, so I continued dating the other guy. My birthday rolled around, April sixth, and a beautiful flower arrangement arrived for me. I knew there was no way these gorgeous flowers were from the guy I was seeing – he was young and poor like me! I read the card and to my surprise they were from Mark!

I called to thank him, and from that moment on, we talked every day. Our first official date was to go see the movie *Beetlejuice* and have dinner at Chili's. (Now, whenever we drive to Baton Rouge, we have to pass that Chili's, and we always point it out, and say, "There's where we had our first date!")

For me, it was definitely love at first sight, but it took Mark a bit longer. He did finally confess that he was interested from the moment he first saw me, but was concerned about asking me out because he was my mom's boss. He could've just fired her. (*Just kidding, Mom!*) We got engaged the following year on my birthday…okay, first there was actually some nonsense where Mark asked me to live with him because he never wanted to get married. My response was, "Fine, I'm moving to Atlanta with a couple of friends. So, see ya!" He suddenly became the marrying kind and proposed with a gorgeous one-carat marquise diamond ring, which I of course accepted.

We planned our wedding for January 27, 1990, which also happened to be the same date my parents were married. It fell on a Saturday and we all agreed that it would be very special to have the same anniversary.

I'd love to say everything leading up to our wedding went perfectly, but this is where things take a turn. In January 1989, Mark's mother Cookie was diagnosed with a brain tumor. She was only 63, had no insurance, and no one to care for her. Mark had moved her to Baton Rouge from Arizona when he found out she was ill. She received medical care at Charity Hospital in New Orleans, but after her brain tumor was removed she needed 24/7 care. Mark found a nursing home in Baton Rouge that accepted Medicaid and moved her there. The brain tumor had affected her memory; I didn't know then about dementia, but that is how she presented. She even wandered out of the nursing home one day, which triggered a huge search party for her. Thankfully, she was found a couple of hours later, happily sitting under a tree. It became part of my routine to stop by every day after work to check on Cookie, and I truly enjoyed spending time with her.

Then in July 1989, Mark received a call from his ex-sister-in-law, that his brother Guy had been killed in a car accident. He was only 36. Mark was devastated.

As we were still grieving this tragic news, my dad suffered a heart attack and died on October 28, 1989. He was 50 years old. I am forever heartbroken that I lost my wonderful father at such a young age.

We weren't done with bad news though. Cookie died a month to the day after my dad on November 28, 1989. She was 64.

We were reeling from the loss of our beloved family members, but decided not to postpone our wedding, which was fast approaching in January. I'm glad we didn't change it, because it gave us a happy event to look forward to.

Mark told me on many occasions, "If we can get through this together, we can get through anything."

I've thought of that often, because life has thrown us a lot of challenges during our 34 years of marriage. In full transparency, there were a few times when we came very close to throwing in the towel, but we stayed together. That's love and commitment.

After our wedding, we decided that we wanted to have a baby right away. We'd had so much loss, it was time for new life. This would be the beginning of one of the most difficult chapters in our lives.

Our journey with infertility could be its own book. In fact, my daughter has told me many times to write about it, and maybe I will one day. It took almost seven years, but finally we were blessed with two beautiful children through the miracle of adoption. Chris, adopted in 1996 from Ecuador, South America, and Abby, adopted in 2003 from Korea. I have always told them both that they were meant to be our children, they just came to us in a different way. I thank God every day that I am Chris and Abby's mom. They are by far the best thing that has ever happened to Mark and me. We have had the greatest time being their parents.

Of course, throughout our marriage, there have been good times and bad. We've made it through job loss, depression issues, and major disagreements. But there have also been many good times, lots of laughter, memorable trips…and through it all, a deep love for each other and our children.

I share all of this, because I think it's important that you know our story.

When people tell me that Mark and I have been so strong through his stroke and the recovery process, I truly believe that all of these losses and challenges we've gone through have made us stronger people.

My belief is that God prepared us for what was to come. He knew it would be our most difficult challenge to date.

CHAPTER 3

From Bad to Worse

The next two days, December 27th and 28th, were a blur for me. Doctors and nurses were in and out of Mark's room. They would take him periodically for one scan or another. I was constantly texting with my kids, my brother Craig, and friend Kathy. Physically, I felt in shock, nauseous, and every fiber of my body felt tense and clenched, especially my jaw. This physical symptom is still with me over a year later. I've learned that under stress I clench my jaw in a big way.

Mark was completely out of it. He would start thrashing in the bed, groaning, and crying out. He was unable to respond to me at all. I asked the medical staff if he was in pain, but I never truly got an answer from anyone. I believe he was. Periodically, I would have to leave the ICU and walk around the hospital. There were Christmas trees and music playing, which felt surreal. To me and the kids, Christmas had come to an abrupt end on December 25th at 7:00 p.m.

It was freezing cold and windy outside. I would go to where the parking garage was and open the door and just stand there, letting the cold wind whip through me. It would give me the jolt I needed to clear my head. Then back to ICU, where I would have to press a buzzer and have someone let me back in. I'd return to my uncomfortable chair to watch over my critically ill husband.

Around midnight of the 27th, Mark began making awful sounds that I have never heard anyone make. To be honest a lot of this I have blocked out of my memory, but I do remember calling Craig, who answered on the first ring. I was still in the room with Mark, so I quietly told him that I thought Mark was going to die. I honestly believe he was very close to death, and I was terrified. Craig told me that he and his wife Dianne would be leaving early in the morning to drive from their home in Gulfport, Mississippi, to be with us in Dallas. I felt such a rush of relief.

I vividly remember at one point through that long night, thinking I NEED AN ADULT and then realizing that I was the adult. Fifty-eight years old, but I didn't feel like an adult in that moment. *I felt like a scared little child.*

Also, during this time I started thinking about the older adults I serve through my business. I've talked to many through the years, whose spouses were in ICU due to a stroke, fall, or other illness. Many times they were in their upper 80's, going through it alone. I couldn't imagine being 85 and going through what I was currently experiencing. It made me so sad. In that moment, the seed for this book was planted. I started typing notes in my iPhone about what it sounded and felt like in the ICU and how scared I was.

Morning finally came and Mark settled down, his condition thankfully improving somewhat. My dear neighbor Sole returned to give me a break. I drove home feeling completely numb. I showered and then tried to lay down in bed for a nap, but I couldn't sleep. Food had no appeal either. I returned to the hospital where Mark had become quite restless again and was thrashing around in his bed. I hugged Sole and thanked her for being there for my family.

That night I resumed my lonely walks through the empty hospital. Around 3 a.m., my back was aching and I just wanted to lie down for a few minutes. I walked out to the abandoned ICU waiting room. The TV was on, and I noticed they had chairs that could be made into sort of a makeshift bed.

I returned to the ICU to get my blanket and then decided to lie down for twenty minutes in one of these "beds" in the waiting room. The lights were on and very bright so I grabbed a face mask and repurposed it as an eye mask. I was feeling quite pleased with my makeshift eye mask, and within five minutes felt myself relaxing a bit, until my peace was rudely interrupted by a male voice, saying, "Ma'am? You can't sleep here." I pulled my face mask from my eyes to see a police officer standing over me. "I'm not sleeping," I responded. "I'm just trying to relax for a few minutes." He started peppering me with questions, apparently they have a problem with homeless people coming in to sleep in the hospital waiting rooms. Once, I proved to him that I was not a homeless woman who had wandered off the streets, and that my husband was indeed in ICU, he left me, but with the strict warning that I couldn't lie down. *You seriously can't make this stuff up.*

There was a recliner in the waiting room, so I sat in it and curled up with my blanket. The TV channel was tuned to some televangelist program and the volume was blaring. I initially felt annoyed. I don't recall what he was saying, but as I listened I started to feel a peace come over me. I knew it was going to be a long road to recovery for Mark, but I also knew that he was going to survive. Just then Abby, my little night owl, called me. I told her about the police officer and the televangelist. My spirits lifted as I talked to her. She and Chris had not seen Mark since his stroke on Christmas Day. It was now December 28th. In some ways it felt like weeks had passed.

By early afternoon on December 28th, the doctors decided that Mark had stabilized enough to leave ICU and go to a regular hospital room. At this point, his right side was completely paralyzed and he was bedridden. The right side of his face drooped, and he couldn't speak. He was having trouble with swallowing and needed two packets of thickeners added to any fluids he drank, and he was also on a pureed food diet.

Mark's neurologist visited and gave us some answers to what caused his strokes. His left carotid artery was blocked, he would need to see a vascular surgeon to find out if there was any surgical recourse, but the blockage, in addition to high blood pressure had broken off plaque which had caused the strokes. The strokes had hit the communication center in his brain, causing *Apraxia* (difficulty with motor planning and coordinating the movements necessary for speech) and *Aphasia* (impairment of expressive language). He also had right sided paralysis, *Hemiplegia*. His neurologist said that Mark would start physical therapy, occupational therapy, and speech therapy while in the hospital, and his next stop would be an in-hospital rehab, followed by long-term rehab. As scary as it was to know the damage the stroke had done, it was encouraging to have a plan in place and feel that we were going to start moving forward.

Craig and Dianne had arrived by this time and Mark was so happy to see them – he burst into tears when they walked into his hospital room. In our entire marriage, I've only seen Mark tear up a few times, but never burst into tears. What a relief to have family with us. It had been a long three days, and I'd had maybe one hour of sleep the entire time. Exhaustion was hitting hard. I drove back home to shower and was finally able to take a nice long nap.

Feeling refreshed, I returned to the hospital bringing Chris and Abby with me. I tried my best to prepare them for how Mark looked (the right side of his face drooped), and sounded- his speech was completely garbled. I'm sure it was frightening for them, but they hugged and kissed him and told him how much they loved him. I know he was happy to see them too.

Things definitely were looking up when Mark played one of his practical jokes on Craig. They were watching a movie, I think it was *Terminator*. Craig was standing on the left side of Mark's hospital bed, and completely engrossed in the film. During a tense moment in the movie, Mark reached over with his left hand and pinched Craig on the butt, causing him to jump and let out a startled yell. Mark was delighted and had a good laugh at Craig's expense.

It was good for all of us to see that Mark's personality was intact – practical jokes and all.

It was getting late and Craig and Dianne had been with Mark most of the day, plus they were getting hungry. They took Chris and Abby with them, but before returning home they stopped at our favorite Mexican restaurant, Mi Día, for dinner and margaritas for everyone. I know the kids were so thankful for that dinner and for their company. I will be forever grateful to them for being there and taking Chris and Abby out for a moment of normalcy.

On the positive side, the new hospital room was much more comfortable and less stressful then the ICU. There was even a couch that made a surprisingly comfortable bed. The bad news, however, was that Mark was extremely agitated and kept trying to pull out his IV…with his teeth!!

I had to keep pressing the buzzer for help, and he would become angry and yell at me, trying to grab it from me using his left hand. His words were slurred, but I had a pretty good idea of what he was trying to convey. At some point the medical team decided to give him something that was supposed to calm him down, but it had the opposite effect. Now, he was trying to pull out his catheter too.

It was non-stop and I quite honestly could not believe this was happening. Despite my best efforts he did pull his IV out using his teeth. I think everyone was horrified. They put it back in and taped it securely to his arm and then gave him another medication that finally knocked him out.

Early the next morning a different doctor came in and he was quite intent on discharging Mark from the hospital. I explained that he had just been moved to this room from ICU. We hadn't even heard from Mark's assigned case manager – we actually never did hear from her, even after I left several messages. There was a picture of her in Mark's room, and Craig recognized her in the hallway one day. He chased her down and told her he was Mark's brother-in-law, and we needed her help. Unfortunately, she still provided us with zero help in finding the best in-hospital rehab for Mark's needs. I would like to say this was an isolated incident, but we experienced more of the same at the next hospital Mark was admitted to for rehab.

I'm not going to sugarcoat it, there is something very wrong with our healthcare system and insurance. I will talk more about this in later chapters.

Unfortunately, timing was not working out for scheduling Mark's move to the rehab hospital. It was the week between Christmas and New Year's, and lots of people were on vacation. We needed to not only figure out which rehab hospital he was going to, and get him approved…but we also had new insurance going into effect on January 1st.

Mr. Mean doctor came back the next morning and again said we needed to leave. *I mean seriously?!* I was so done with him, that I told him to leave the room. My sister-in-law Dianne was so outraged by how this doctor was treating me, that she relayed to Mark's neurologist what was going on. He was not pleased and apparently spoke with the mean doctor. We didn't see him again, which was good, because Mark didn't receive insurance approval to move to the rehab hospital until January 5th!

Craig and Dianne returned to Mississippi on December 30th. We were all sad to see them go, but thankful for the time we had them with us. It definitely helped to have family there with me, especially Dianne with her medical knowledge. I felt better and more at peace with the decisions I had made on Mark's behalf.

During our long wait to move to the rehab, Chris started coming to the hospital in the evening to stay with Mark, so I could go home and get some much needed rest. He would arrive every night at seven p.m. Chris is an interesting guy, he doesn't care what anyone thinks of him, which is a wonderful trait to have. He's on the autism spectrum, although very high functioning. Each night, he would arrive wearing pajamas, slippers and carrying his pillow. The door to Mark's room would fly open and he would announce, "I'm here!" It was hilariously funny and classic Christopher. He and Mark settled into a routine of watching one Marvel movie each night and then they'd go to sleep.

It still brings tears to my eyes to remember walking into Mark's room in the early morning and seeing Chris tending to his dad – brushing his teeth, adjusting his bed or adding thickeners to his juice. Chris has continued to show what a natural caregiver he is throughout Mark's recovery. I honestly don't know what I would've done without his help.

I am so thankful that I had several friends providing guidance on the best rehab for Mark. I ended up choosing one in Dallas, although in retrospect, I wish I had gone with my gut instinct and moved him to one that was closer to my house.

Insurance approved his transfer on January 5th, and the next step was to wait for an ambulance to transfer him to the hospital rehab. I was sitting with him in his hospital room waiting on the ambulance to arrive, when he suddenly became very agitated. I couldn't understand what he was saying, but suddenly pillows were being flung at my head with surprising accuracy. Fortunately, at that moment the nurse walked in to let us know that the ambulance had arrived. She looked at the pillows on the floor, and the look on my face, but didn't say a word. The timing was perfect as the gurney was rolled in. I was happy for the brief break I would get as Mark was transported by ambulance, and I followed behind.

There was a sense of relief as we said goodbye to this hospital where our lives had been turned upside down, and hello to the rehab hospital. In this next chapter of recovery, Mark would start receiving the intense rehab needed to hopefully get back all that the strokes had stolen from him.

From this point on, Mark would be in rehabs until mid-July.

As I write this, it's still hard to believe that one minute we were about to sit down to enjoy our Christmas dinner and in the next, Mark would suffer four debilitating strokes and not return home for almost seven months.

CHAPTER 4

What is a Stroke?

Basically, a stroke, also called a CVA or cerebrovascular accident, causes **damage** to the brain by interrupting blood supply. There are two main types of strokes:

- **Ischemic** – this is the most common (about 87% of all strokes according to the Center for Disease control, CDC), and was the type of stroke Mark had. This type of stroke happens when a blood vessel supplying blood to your brain becomes blocked by a blood clot or piece of plaque. The two most common causes are due to atherosclerosis (narrowing of arteries due to plaque buildup) or atrial fibrillation (aFib).
  Mark's strokes were due to atherosclerosis and pieces of plaque that had broken off.
- **Hemorrhagic** – happens when there is bleeding in the brain. Causes include high blood pressure, an aneurysm, or vascular malformation.

I saw Mark's MRI of his brain after his strokes; there were four purple dots, which were indicators of where the strokes were. Those spots on his brain are now *permanently damaged.* It took me a little time to absorb and process that fact as I stared at his MRI.

It's also important to note that if the stroke occurs on the left side of the brain, it affects the right side of the body and vice versa. This is because each side of the brain controls the opposite side of the body. Mark's strokes were on the left side of his brain, which is why his right side was affected.

Now, the good news is that our brains are pretty incredible and through something called **neuroplasticity** can essentially reroute around the damaged areas. By the way, I did NOT know this word prior to Mark's strokes, but I know it well now – and can even spell it!

What is neuroplasticity? It's the ability of neural networks in the brain to change through growth and reorganization and create new pathways. Mark's neurologist said something very similar to me, but then he saw my utter look of confusion and explained it this way, which makes perfect sense…

You're driving down the road and you come to a roadblock. The road is not passable so you're stuck, but then you see a detour sign. You follow the detour sign around the roadblock and you're on your way. The stroke has caused a roadblock in your brain, so you have to create a detour – that is neuroplasticity!

Ta-da! Makes sense, right?

The way to create the detours is through lots and lots of repetition through Physical Therapy, Occupational Therapy, and Speech Therapy. It's all about rehab AND mindset. We will talk more about mindset in a later chapter.

Strokes are, sadly, quite common, and it is a leading cause of death for Americans. I pulled some alarming statistics from the CDC website (cdc.gov).

- In 2021, one in six deaths from cardiovascular disease was due to stroke.
- Every 40 seconds, someone in the US has a stroke. Every three minutes and fourteen seconds, someone dies of stroke.
- Every year, more than 795,000 people in the US have a stroke. About 610,000 of these are first or new strokes.
- About 185,000 strokes – nearly one in four – are in people who have had a previous stroke.
- About 87% of all strokes are ischemic strokes, in which blood flow to the brain is blocked.
- Stroke is a leading cause of serious long-term disability. Stroke reduces mobility in more than half of stroke survivors age 65 and older.

Scary right? Like a lot of people, I thought strokes were something that happened to older people. I have met many people on this journey whose loved one had a stroke in their

20's, 30's, 40's and 50's. Honestly, no age is immune from suffering a stroke. In fact, according to the CDC… **"stroke risk increases with age, but strokes can – and do – occur at any age."**

How about this sobering statistic, also from the CDC:

In 2014, **38%** of people hospitalized for stroke were **less than 65 years old**.

Now that I've been a Debbie Downer, let's talk about the causes of stroke and how to PREVENT them!

Most strokes are preventable (70-80%) and that's encouraging news. We all have risk factors that are within our control and others that are not. The American Stroke Association (www.stroke.org) has an incredible website that you should visit, but following are the highlights.

Risk Factors we CANNOT control:

- Age – likelihood of a stroke goes up as we age
- Family History – if a family member had a stroke, especially before age 65
- Race – black people have a much higher risk of death from a stroke
- Gender – women have more strokes than men and are more likely to die from the stroke
- Prior Stroke, TIA, or Heart Attack

Risk Factors we CAN control:

- High Blood Pressure – know your numbers! Optimal blood pressure is less than 120/80
- Smoking – DON'T! 58.8% of stroke survivors in the US were smokers
- Diabetes
- Diet
- Physical Inactivity
- Obesity
- High Cholesterol - again, know your numbers! Have your cholesterol checked regularly and if it can't be controlled through diet, discuss statin medications with your doctor
- Atrial Fibrillation (AFib) – heart rhythm disorder (there is medical treatment for this)
- Sleep Apnea – more than half of the people who have a stroke, also have sleep apnea

KNOWING THE SIGNS OF A STROKE

It's important for everyone to know the signs of a stroke. I mentioned earlier that I knew Mark was having a stroke because of a commercial I had seen many years ago called FAST. For some reason it always stayed with me, which is why I knew immediately that Mark was having a stroke.

The acronym is FAST, and here is the breakdown:

F – Face (Ask the person to smile. Does one side droop?)
A – Arms (Ask the person to raise both arms. Does one arm drift downward?)
S – Speech (Ask the person to repeat a simple sentence. Are the words slurred?)
T – Time (If the person shows any of these symptoms, call 911 immediately!)

With his first stroke, the only sign was speech for Mark. He was slurring and unable to remember a blessing he had said probably thousands of times. His strokes in the ICU were different, his face immediately drooped to the right, as did his entire body. When the medical staff came in to assess him, his smile drooped on the right side, he could not lift his right arm and his speech was not only slurred, but made no sense.

Also, learn from the mistake I made during Mark's first stroke at home…when it comes to Time, all I could focus on was getting him medical help FAST. I should have called 911. I took Mark to the closest hospital, but unfortunately they did not specialize in Neurology, and he had to be taken by CareFlite to a hospital 30 minutes away. If I had called 911, the ambulance would've transported him to a different hospital that specialized in neurology, saving us time and money.

Sidenote: You aren't going to believe how much that helicopter transport ended up costing me. I'll address that later when I talk about Healthcare and Insurance.

CHAPTER 5

How Best to Help a Family in Crisis

Sharing the news of a loved one's catastrophic illness or accident is a very personal decision.

The night of Mark's stroke, after I got him to the Emergency Room, I called my brother, my mom, and our neighbors Marco and Sole. I also messaged Mark's brother Karl who lives in California. The next day, once I knew more about what was going on, I posted what had happened on Facebook. I was comfortable with this mode of communication because I am very active on social media. Mark and I use it to stay connected with family and friends who live all of over the United States, as well as with friends and family who live overseas.

I am also a huge believer in prayer, and I wanted as many people as I could get praying for Mark.

Prayers and messages began flowing in immediately, which brought such comfort for all of us. We could feel the love and prayers all around us.

Everyone wanted to help, which was wonderful, however they all had the same questions…

What do you need?
What can I do?

I know these questions came from the purest place in their hearts, and certainly I would be asking the same questions if I were in their position.

However, I learned something interesting about the human mind. When you are stressed and overwhelmed to the level I was, you honestly have no idea how to respond. My mind was a complete blank. All I could think to say was please just pray for Mark and for Chris and Abby.

Well, I am so thankful that my friends all flew into action, and there will never be words to express our gratitude for all they did for us.

I think it's important to share here in a list format, because I believe it can be helpful to others who may want to help a friend or family member going through a crisis. These are some of the ways people helped us:

1. <u>Provide Meals</u> – The thought of preparing meals, or even if there was food in the refrigerator did not even register in my thoughts. One of the ladies who works for me, Sarah (or "Sweet Sarah" as we all call her), texted me to see if I was okay with her setting up a Meal Train. Of course I was! She quickly put the Meal Train together with our likes, allergies, etc., and put it on Facebook. Dates immediately filled up. Sarah told me later that she had to keep adding more dates, because so many people wanted to bring us a meal. We ended up with meals for a month, plus DoorDash and Restaurant Gift Cards mailed to us or slid under our front doormat. I was absolutely amazed, as were Chris and Abby. It was such a relief to know that the kids had food and that when I returned home from the hospital at 8:00 p.m., there was always something delicious to eat.

2. <u>Send a Card</u> – A simple card just knowing that our friends and family were thinking of us and praying meant the world to us. As most of our friends know, we are obsessed with our golden retriever Sadie, and many of the cards we received featured golden retrievers. Later, when Mark was in rehab, I taped all of the cards to his wall and it cheered him up immensely.

3. <u>Offer to Walk the Dog or Care for Pets</u> – So many people offered to do this for us, and I thought it was such a generous offer. Thankfully, Chris was home and caring for all three of our dogs, but I

definitely would've needed help with this if we didn't have family to help.

4. <u>Lunch Bag and Diet Coke</u> – This one needs some explaining. While at the hospital, I had posted a picture on Facebook of a Diet Pepsi, and my total despair that it was not a Diet Coke. I think all hospitals in Texas carry Pepsi products only, not sure why that is. Later that day I returned home to find the cutest lunch bag, with a six-pack of Diet Coke and freezer packs to keep it cool. Such a thoughtful gift from a friend.

5. <u>Pack up Christmas Decorations</u> – Mark had his stroke on Christmas Day and unfortunately I had decided to make 2022 the year that Christmas exploded all over our house. I had three trees and decorations everywhere. As I mentioned before, Christmas ended for all of us at seven p.m. Christmas Day. It was actually depressing for me, Chris, and Abby to see the house festively decorated. I wasn't home much, and when I was, it was only to eat and catch a few hours of sleep. My friend Joie has a moving company, and she brought her team over one day while I was at the hospital with Mark. They packed up all of my decorations and organized my Christmas closet, and believe me it was in major need of organizing! They did a fantastic job, and when I came home that evening the sheer relief made me cry happy tears. I am forever grateful to her and her team for this act of kindness.

6. <u>Clean out the Garage</u> – My friend Aricia was concerned about how I would get Mark out of the car and in through the garage when he returned home. A valid concern, but not one I'd had time to consider. Let's just say Mark is a "collector" of tools and other manly garage items. Aricia organized a group of neighbors and friends to meet at my house one Saturday morning. We all worked for several hours clearing out the garage, getting rid of junk, adding peg board to hold tools and organizing the rest into bins. I'm not sure my garage had ever looked this good, and it knocked one more thing off my to-do list.

7. <u>GoFundMe</u> – This was a tough one for me to agree to, but it was necessary. We were quickly accumulating a mountain of medical debt, although we had insurance, our coverage in 2022 was through a Medi-Share plan, which I will go into more detail about later in the book. Also, as time progressed and I began to understand that Mark would very likely be permanently disabled, I had to have a bathroom remodeled to fit his needs. A group of friends got together and created a GoFundMe for Mark. I was overwhelmed by how many people donated, and it definitely has helped with some of the expenses we have incurred.

8. <u>Fundraisers</u> – Several friends also had fundraisers for Mark at restaurants, stores, and through their home-businesses. We will never forget their kindness and generosity.

9. <u>Fix things around the house</u> – I'm not good at asking for help, but I have to confess I am not super handy. Although, I have learned through YouTube how to fix two toilet issues, and I fixed my gate temporarily by tying it closed with orange ribbon – thank you to my neighbor Sole for supplying the ribbon and laughs! There were a few things I couldn't fix and my neighbors and Abby's boyfriend Zane (who is a plumber!) were happy to help.

10. <u>Gift a Massage</u> – One dear friend not only gifted me a massage, but even asked me to let her know the day I was going so she could call and leave the tip. So sweet. Over the past year, I've been gifted by friends with massage gift certificates. Stress as the caregiver is real, and I appreciate such a thoughtful gift.

11. <u>Prayer</u> – The most important. I have family and friends of all different faiths and beliefs. We soaked in all of their prayers, good energy, positive thoughts, all that was offered for Mark's healing was much appreciated.

I'm sure there are many other ways to help a friend in need. Just remember, they may not be able to articulate an answer to the question – *What can I do for you?* Be prepared to jump into action with some of the things mentioned above.

I'd also like to add a few items on what NOT to say to someone going through this type of crisis.

- "I guess you're out of business now." Someone actually said this when we were on Day Three of Mark's medical crisis. What is the point of saying something like this? My business supports my family, it pays for the insurance that is covering the medical bills for Mark's care. I am thankful that I am self-employed and that I have an amazing team. We did not miss a beat, and by the time Mark was out of ICU, I had my laptop and was working between doctors and nurses coming in and out of the room. I can't imagine what would've happened if I'd had a regular job to go to everyday. I'm sure I would've been fired.

- "My heart hurts for Mark that you are using traditional medicine. You should use my supplements." I would love to tell you that I'm joking, but an acquaintance seriously messaged me this on Facebook. I had a lot of pent up rage that was released in my response to her.

- "This has all really aged you." Ummm, please just don't say this to anyone, especially a 58-year-old woman. I'm sure stress and lack of sleep had me not looking my best, but did someone really need to say this to me?

- "I have exciting news. Since you're so busy with Mark, I'm starting a business just like yours, in the same town." From an acquaintance. I'm truly not sure what the proper response to this would have been, but I think she expected me to be happy and congratulate her.

CHAPTER 6

Insurance, Hospitals, and CareFlite

The topic of health insurance and hospitals kind of throws me into a blind rage at this point, but I do want to share my experience in the hope of helping others. I'm sure this will come as no surprise to anyone, but navigating through the medical system in our country is a nightmare.

I'm self-employed, which automatically limits healthcare options. In December 2022, we had a Medi-Share plan. This is not true health insurance; it's basically a large group of people who pay monthly and share in the payment of eligible medical bills. It's more of a catastrophic plan. To claim a medical "incident" it has to be over $500, and you must request the "cash" or "uninsured" price for all medical procedures, doctors, hospitals, etc. It can take up to six months to receive payment from the Medi-Share plan, and it is not guaranteed.

We had successfully used it several years ago, when Mark had an emergency appendectomy.

In November of 2022, I had an uneasy, gut feeling about this plan. I felt like we needed to get real insurance, although we were limited to the Exchange (ObamaCare), which are all HMO's. Mark was against this idea. He was of the belief, and I've since learned that many other people believe this as well, that if you get sick the hospital has to take care of you. Well, the answer to that is yes and no. They will save your life, but good luck getting the rehab you may need to recover any quality of life.

I simply couldn't shake the feeling that we needed true insurance, so I called a friend who sells all types of insurance plans and she pulled together a few Blue Cross Blue Shield (BCBS) plans from the Exchange. They were expensive and I reviewed them with Mark or tried to, but he was adamant that we were fine with the Medi-Share plan.

I have learned throughout my life to pay attention to gut feelings, so on December 15, 2022, I signed up for the BCBS exchange plan and scheduled it to go into effect on January 1, 2023. Thank God I listened to my intuition.

From 12/25/22 through 12/31/22, Mark was covered under the Medi-Share Plan. They did cover much of the expenses, but not all. The problem we would have run into if BCBS had not gone into effect on 1/1/23 is with the rehab hospital. They were requesting I pay them in advance – they would NOT accept the Medi-Share plan. Let me be clear, they wanted $80,000 up front.

Time was on our side, because of the delay in moving forward between Christmas and New Year's, Mark wasn't transferred to the rehab hospital until 1/5/23 and by that time the BCBS plan was fully in effect. Whew!

Here's the truly scary thing – if I did not have insurance do you think Mark would have been accepted into rehab? No.

I have since talked to many, self-employed, successful business people in their 50's who do not have healthcare of any kind. *Y'all, please get insurance, because I am having a mini panic attack on your behalf.*

I know how limited and expensive the options are, but the BCBS HMO plan I bought on the exchange has covered ALL of Mark's rehab. They are still at this time paying for outpatient neuro rehab five days a week. He has been receiving some form of rehab for over a year now. Without access to this intense rehab that he is still receiving, he would not be recovered to the point he is today.

Hospitals.

We need them, of course, and there are many wonderful and caring people who work in them. My question though, is how is it possible that a two-hour Emergency Room visit can cost $24,000? That is the cash or uninsured price. Most hospitals are in the business of making money, I get that, but doesn't this seem extreme?

I did my very best to be responsible and have insurance coverage for my family, but even with a Medi-Share plan and an HMO, the medical bills have been overwhelming. The medical debt continues to add up as Mark has had additional testing and hospitalizations.

I don't have the answers for how to fix our healthcare system, but I can testify to the fact that it is very broken. I'm not a political person at all, but I pray that one day both sides will find a way to agree and come up with a plan to help the American people they love to say they care so much about.

Let's talk about CareFlite. This may be called something different depending on where you live. It's emergency helicopter transportation. A much needed service clearly, and I'm thankful they were there to transport Mark to the hospital where he could receive the stroke care he needed.

However, no one mentioned that this service was going to cost $35,130 – and that collection calls would begin almost immediately – in our case Mark's fourth day in the hospital. I remember clearly because he had just been moved to a regular room.

CareFlite does not set up payment plans; they want the entire $35,130 paid in full immediately.

Also, just to make it clear, I did not request that CareFlite come pick up my husband and transport him. I actually had many people ask me why I had Mark airlifted to the second hospital. This was NOT a choice that I made. If you've not been in this situation, and I hope you never are, here's how it happened.

The first time I heard the word CareFlite was in the ER at the first hospital when the nurse came in and said, *"CareFlite is 20 minutes out."* Of course, it's not like I was going to say, "Wait! How much is this going to cost?" Or "Just throw him in the back of my car and I'll drive him to the hospital."

When your loved one is critically ill, you place all of your trust in the doctors who are caring for them. If the doctor believes the best shot is CareFlite because time is of the essence, you are not going to argue.

I remember afterwards joking with my brother about how much the bill was going to be. I think we were guessing around $10,000. When I received the bill of $35,130 – I nearly needed medical attention myself.

It took several months, but thankfully the Medi-Share plan did pay the bill in its entirety. The way it works with Medi-Share plans, is they send you a check and then you pay the bill.

Sidenote: I have had a few people tell me that there is some kind of insurance you can purchase in advance from CareFlite.

CHAPTER 7

The Role of Advocate for Your Loved One

No one is ever prepared for a loved one's sudden health crisis. When it happens, we are not only in shock, but we may also be thrust into the role of being their advocate and trying to navigate through a system we don't understand.

My dad had been hospitalized for almost a week after he had his heart attack in 1989. I remember he was in ICU and honestly he didn't look too bad to me. My dad was my hero, and I thought he was invincible. He was on oxygen which concerned me, but he was still joking around, and even asked me to go get him a burger and chocolate shake from Burger King. I said no, obviously, because he had just had a heart attack! He died the next day, so I do have some regret that I didn't get him the damn junk food he was craving.

My mom was in charge, talking to the doctors, being a total Rockstar as his advocate. I don't remember much about what tests were being run on him, and it's very likely that I didn't even ask. At 25 years old, and three months shy of my wedding day, there was no way I could imagine him not being okay. I thought maybe he'd need surgery, but he'd recover in time to walk me down the aisle. Unfortunately, his heart was so damaged that there was nothing they could do, and he died in the hospital on October 28, 1989.

As I sat next to Mark's hospital bed awaiting approval for the next step in his journey, I thought a lot about my dad. I couldn't imagine Mark not surviving this, our kids were only 26 and 19. I knew the total devastation of losing a parent at their age, and I prayed they would not have to experience it. I also thought about my mom, and how she had stayed by my dad's side the entire time he was in the hospital. I remember her telling me that during his last night, probably hours before he died, he told her, *"I love you with my whole bad heart."*

I am a very determined person, and decided right then that I would make sure Mark had the very best care and we would do everything possible to help him make a full recovery. I remember telling the kids that we were going to stay positive, I think this is when we also came up with #TeamWilliams, which I included on many of my social media posts. A bit cheesy maybe, but it motivated us which was the goal.

Mark needed an advocate and, by gosh, I was going to be the best damn advocate ever!

It definitely helped that my background is in senior living, and I had helped many people navigate through hospitals and rehabs due to strokes or other illnesses. I knew the terminology too, which was a benefit. Plus, I had lots of friends who worked in healthcare standing by to help in any way that they could.

I realize how much having this knowledge helped me, and sharing this information is one of the main reasons I'm writing this book.

*   *   *   *   *

In the following section, I'm going to share the process or steps involved after a sudden illness or accident. I will use Mark's stroke as an example. I will also breakdown the basic terminology you are likely to encounter as an advocate for your loved one.

When a patient first arrives at the hospital either by ambulance or walk-in, the first thing will be to stabilize and assess them. Next, depending on the severity of their illness or injury, they may be sent to *ICU (Intensive Care Unit)*. Once they're no longer deemed critical, the patient is moved to a regular hospital room. At this point, you should have the name of the *case manager* who has been assigned to your loved one. The case manager will help you with *discharge planning*, which is developing a plan for appropriate services and support that will be needed upon discharge. This could mean transitioning to a rehabilitation center, assisted living, outpatient therapy, or home with services.

Following are the steps we went through for Mark's care:

- Emergency Room at the first hospital – Mark was stabilized, assessed, and it was determined he was having a stroke. They then consulted with their sister hospital that had a neurology department and determined the best option was to begin treatment with the clot-busting medication, Tenecteplase. He was deemed critical, and transported by helicopter to the second hospital's Emergency Room, and then admitted to their ICU.

- On the fourth day of his stay, he was stable enough to be moved to a regular hospital room. His rehab was started at this time, with *Physical Therapy, Occupational Therapy,* and *Speech Therapy.*

- The neurologist recommended that Mark be discharged to an *in-hospital rehabilitation*, also known as acute rehabilitation or inpatient rehabilitation. This type of rehab is designed for patients who have experienced severe injuries, surgeries, illnesses, or conditions such as strokes, and is in a hospital setting, as the patient still requires close medical supervision, in addition to intensive rehabilitation. The rehab is usually three hours per day. The patient will also be assigned a case manager. In Mark's case, he stayed ten days at an in-hospital rehab in Dallas. Living in a large metropolitan area, we had many options to choose from. My main goal was to find one that specialized in stroke recovery. Mark arrived in an ambulance on a gurney. After intense rehab, he left for his next stop in a wheelchair.

Note: this may not be the next step for everyone. Many people are discharged from the hospital to a Skilled Nursing Facility (SNF) for rehab. They continue to receive nursing care plus Physical Therapy, Occupational Therapy and Speech Therapy, but not at the some intense level as provided in an in-hospital rehab. Average stay is typically seven-to-ten days. Most people would then return to their home or, depending on their diagnosis, may be better served by moving into senior housing.

- Mark's next step was to be admitted into a *live-in rehabilitation treatment center* that provided specialized brain injury and stroke rehabilitation. I chose Pate Brain Injury and Stroke Rehabilitation. They have three sites, but the one that appealed to me the most was Brinlee Creek Ranch in Anna, Texas. It was a long drive from my house, but I felt the quiet, country setting would be healing, and I knew Mark would prefer the country over the city. Plus, they had two donkeys and a horse!

- *Outpatient Neuro Rehabilitation* – From what I understand, this is not available everywhere, but living in a large metropolitan area like Dallas, we had a couple of good options to choose from. We chose the Centre for Neuro Skills in Irving for

Mark. It's only fifteen minutes from our house, and Mark goes to rehab four hours a day, five days a week. Transportation is even provided. This is covered by our insurance and his progress is reviewed each month to determine continued eligibility. He continues to make progress, so hopefully he will remain enrolled in this rehab for a long time.

- *In-Home Therapy* – Once home, your loved one will likely continue in rehab either outpatient or in their home. This is not just for stroke recovery, but for hip replacement, recovery from an illness, etc. You can find Physical Therapists, Occupational Therapists and Speech Therapists either through their own businesses or through Home Health Agencies. Insurance will pay for a set number of visits, and must be deemed medically necessary and ordered by a physician.

SPEAK UP!

Remember, as the Advocate for your loved one it's *your* responsibility to speak up and ask questions. Navigating your way through the system can be overwhelming and confusing – not to mention, you're likely sleep deprived and stressed!

I have found that it can be harder for older people to question what the doctor tells them. They grew up in a time where the doctor knew best and you didn't ask questions. You can and should ask questions, especially if you don't understand the information being relayed to you.

I asked LOTS of questions. Most of the doctors were happy to explain to me what was happening in Mark's brain due to his strokes. (Remember, the neurologist who gave me the analogy about a detour when explaining neuroplasticity?)

As the advocate, find out when the doctors/specialists/therapists will be coming by so you can be there for an update about your loved one's condition and to ask any questions that you may have. Most are happy to answer your questions.

Your loved one will be assigned a social worker or case manager to help you with the next steps. Most do an amazing job, as we have experienced at Pate Rehab and the Centre for Neuro Skills.

Unfortunately, we had two negative experiences at two separate hospitals. I shared in an earlier chapter how my brother chased Mark's elusive case manager down the hallway at the first hospital. Even after he spoke with her, she still didn't provide us with assistance. I was able to figure out the next steps for Mark's rehab, because of my previous knowledge working in senior living and my network of healthcare professionals. I can't imagine how lost I would have felt without my experience and relationships.

The worst experience I had with a case manager occurred in the Dallas in-hospital rehab Mark had been transferred to following his discharge from the first hospital. It had a sterling reputation for stroke rehab, and Mark did receive excellent care. However, the case manager assigned to him not only provided zero help, but in my opinion, she went out of her way to be cruel to me.

The rehab was in the Dallas Medical District, which was about a thirty-minute drive from my house, if you didn't go during peak traffic times. I made the drive every single day, but was no longer spending each night at the hospital, for several reasons, most importantly because I was completely physically and emotionally exhausted. Mark was in therapy most of the day, which gave me time to catch up on work.

A conference call was scheduled for an update on how Mark was progressing. On the call were his doctors, therapists, and the case manager. They each took a turn providing an update, and the news was encouraging. The last to speak was the case manager, and her contribution was…*the family is not present to provide support and no personal effects have even been brought to his room.* I was too stunned to speak. One of the therapists spoke up and said there are get well cards and pictures in his room, and I see his wife here every day. By this point, I was on the verge of tears and could only manage to squeak out, yes there are cards and pictures. I don't remember much more about that call, but it ended soon after the awful and untrue words spoken by the case manager.

I was sitting on the couch in my living room. I hung up the phone and I started sobbing uncontrollably. Chris was in the other room and bless his heart he ran to me and grabbed me in a bear hug, saying, "It's okay, Mom." I quickly realized that he thought Mark had died or had another stroke, so I pulled myself together and told him that dad was okay, it was just that the case manager had been very mean to me on the conference call.

This woman went out of her way to say something untrue and hurtful. I felt very judged and honestly after I processed through those feelings, I was enraged. How could someone, especially a case manager, be so awful and add more stress to a person who is already in crisis?

I had planned to contact the hospital after Mark was discharged to relay what had happened, but honestly, I didn't have the energy. We moved forward and got him settled in at Pate Rehab, where he had a wonderful case manager. She was quick to answer questions, compassionate, and even gave me a great resource that helped me with filing for Mark's Social Security Disability.

That is what a case manager is supposed to do.

As the advocate for your loved one, If you feel uncomfortable about a treatment or any member of the care team – *Speak Up!* I wish now that I had spoken up about the treatment I received by the case manager. I'm sure I am not the only victim of her cruelty. I can say this, I would *never* take Mark back to that rehab hospital.

Many Hospitals are understaffed, and in my experience this was very obvious on weekends. Of course, during Mark's stay in the first hospital, the timing was especially difficult. He was there during the holiday week between Christmas and New Year's, which I'm sure made the situation worse. I'm not faulting or judging anyone, just stating a fact.

I was hyper-vigilant when anyone came in to give Mark medications, because the strokes had affected his ability to swallow. His pills all had to be crushed and put in applesauce or pudding for him to take. This was noted on a sign behind his bed, on a dry/erase board on the wall in front of his bed, and I'm sure it was also noted in his file on the computer in his room that was accessed by all medical personnel.

One weekend night, the nurse on duty came to give Mark his medications. I jumped up and yelled, "No!" as I saw her hand Mark a little cup full of uncrushed pills, that he readily accepted with his left hand. I scooped the cup out of his hand, while pointing to the signs in the room that his medications were to be crushed. I shudder to think what would have happened if I hadn't been in the room, and alert to what was going on.

Another issue I caught before it became a serious concern was the beginning of a pressure wound on the heel of Mark's right foot. Because I work in senior living, I knew that lying in bed for an extended period of time, especially not being able to move one side of the body, could lead to pressure wounds. I decided to check Mark's foot and sure enough there was a small red spot forming on his heel, about the size of a dime. I called my sister-in-law who, as I mentioned earlier, is a nurse anesthetist and described to her what I was seeing. She confirmed that it was likely the beginning of a pressure wound. I immediately called for the nurse and they began treatment on his foot.

Again, as the advocate, it's imperative that you are alert to any changes your loved one may experience. If you're thinking, I don't have medical experience or anyone in health care to call and ask about potential issues, you don't have to. Just do your best by staying in the loop with the healthcare providers and keeping an eye out for any changes.

I also tried to always be present when the therapists came in, so I could ask questions and see what exercises they were doing with Mark. I'm so glad I was there to witness the Physical Therapists standing him up for the first time since his strokes. It took two very strong therapists, a gait belt, and a lot of positioning, but they got him up. I was jumping up and down cheering him on. It was such an incredible moment.

When you see someone you love begin to recover from a critical illness, every tiny step they take forward is a huge accomplishment. Early on I decided that we were going to celebrate every single win no matter how small... a win is a win. I became Mark's biggest cheerleader and I still am today!

The therapists were all concerned about the delay in getting Mark to the in-hospital rehab so he could begin intense rehabilitation. We were caught in a tough place, due to the timing and that our insurance wasn't going into effect until January 1st. It was scary because I knew the sooner Mark was moved to the rehab, the better his outcome would be. I asked the therapists to show me and Chris exercises that we could do with him.

We would open his right hand, massaging his fingers so they wouldn't get stuck curled in. Massaged lotion into his right arm and used a soft brush on his arm in hopes of stimulating the nerves. We did exercises with his right foot and leg, moving it up, bending it in. This was a tough one for me, because his leg was heavy! Chris and I became experts in moving Mark up in his bed, he was constantly sliding down, and positioning pillows around him to keep him as comfortable as possible.

Communication is on the left side of the brain, which had been damaged by Mark's strokes resulting in Aphasia and Apraxia. The speech therapist gave us exercises to do with him, including singing "Happy Birthday" and the "ABC's." Mark wasn't always the best patient for me, and would get annoyed and not want to participate. One day, when I had given up on trying to get him to do the speech exercises, I sneezed and he immediately said "Bless You." He said it perfectly.

I was again reminded of how amazing our brains are. Even though the strokes had caused damage to his communication center, rote memories like saying "Bless you!" after someone sneezes are still there.

Also, interestingly enough, most of his curse words were still intact, and he was now using those quite frequently!

CHAPTER 8

The Role of Caregiver

Mark completed his in-hospital rehab in mid-January and was then transferred to an in-patient neuro rehab, Pate Rehab, where he would remain until mid-July. Throughout that time I felt that I moved into the dual role of advocate and caregiver.

Speech remained a challenge for Mark and I could only imagine how frustrating and lonely that must have felt. I asked him if he'd like for me to make a sign for his door with a list of all the things people should know about him. He quickly said yes! On my way home I stopped and bought a sheet of poster board and stickers – it became a bit of a craft project for me. I thought of everything I could about him, that he'd want people to know. On the poster board, I wrote:

> My name is Mark.
> My wife is Lori.
> I have two kids, Chris and Abby.

I have a golden retriever named Sadie.
I love music from the 70's, especially The Beatles.
I worked as Vice President of Operations.

I added a few more facts, decorated it with stickers and then taped it to the door to his room in the rehab. He loved it. I felt like it helped the caregivers connect with him and get to know him as a person. We don't realize how important the ability to communicate is until we lose it.

With a brain injury, which is what a stroke is, there were occasional outbursts of sadness or anger from Mark. As the spouse, unfortunately, you are the one they take it out on. I'm told it's because you are their safe person. Speaking the truth here, it doesn't feel good, especially when you are the person keeping all the balls in the air, your life completely revolves around your ill spouse and on top of everything else, you're sleep deprived and stressed.

I have great empathy for Mark. I can't even begin to comprehend how it would feel not to be able to communicate. His aphasia made his speech extremely difficult to understand. He knew what he wanted to say, but we couldn't understand him.

One day Chris and I were visiting him at rehab. He tried to tell us something and became so angry that he started yelling and motioning for us to go. It was truly awful, but I grabbed my purse and told him goodbye. The rehab was almost an hour from our house. I'm not a crier, but it was taking everything in my power not to burst into tears as I drove away from the rehab. Chris was quiet, and I felt awful for him too. There was a Rockfish restaurant close by, and I steered the car to it. I told Chris we need a stiff drink and a good meal. Even though it helped, I felt a lot of fear about what life would be like when Mark returned home and I would be his full-time caregiver.

To be honest, being a caregiver has never been something I wanted to be. In fact, I'll admit I had some very angry discussions with God about it. Having worked in senior living as long as I have, I've talked to many people who have been caregivers for their family members. I always had great respect and concern for them and always reminded them to take care of themselves.

Now, I'm in the role of caregiver and I can't stand it when someone tells me to take care of myself. I feel more stress when someone tells me that, because it feels like another task being added onto my already overflowing plate. I know I need to take care of myself, but unfortunately the easiest appointments to cancel are the ones for myself. I now understand why caregivers neglect their own health. I was so busy making sure Mark made it to all of his appointments, driving back and forth to his rehab, getting the house ready for his return, running my business, and so much more. The easiest appointments to cancel were mine. The dentist and my annual physical would have to wait.

As things have settled down, and we are in more of a routine, I have caught up on all of my medical appointments. I even have monthly massages and facials at my favorite salon, Lakeside Wellness and Apothecary. Simply walking into the salon soothes my soul. The two lovely ladies I see, and who are both dear friends, are Melissa and Livea, and they have helped me learn more about my body's response to stress and how to use meditation to help relieve it.

Mark was scheduled to be discharged from rehab in mid-August 2023, however, as I was visiting him in mid-July, I was told his discharge date had changed, and he would be going home in three days. I was happy he was coming home, but terrified about becoming his full-time caregiver. Plus, I thought I had another month to prepare. I seriously questioned whether I would be able to work full-time and care for him, and not working was not an option. I was not in a position to retire.

Luckily, I am very proactive by nature, so the house was ready and handicapped accessible. We had brought him home for a couple of weekend stays, and he seemed to be managing well with the modifications we had made to the house.

I wanted to make Mark's return home super special, so I called a local company, Card My Yard, and ordered a huge sign for the yard. The owner was happy to help out with this project, and came up with some great ideas. I told her that we called Mark our superhero, and that it would be awesome if she had cutouts of superheroes, she did. The sign turned out better than I could have imagined. It said, "WELCOME HOME WARRIOR" and had hearts, stars, and superheroes all around it. Mark loved it!

When the day of Mark's discharge arrived, Chris, Abby and I drove out to the rehab to pick him up. The rehab had a really lovely graduation ceremony for him where he actually walked with his cane through a line of therapists all clapping for him. The other patients were also clapping and a few people were even crying, Abby and I included. We loaded the van with all of his belongings, including a bag full of his medications and a list of what to take when. There was A LOT of medicine!

There is definitely an adjustment period when you bring someone home with disabilities. I was now fully immersed in the role of caregiver and feeling a bit overwhelmed. The first few weeks were not easy, as we tried to establish a new routine. Shower time was especially difficult for me, because I had received no training on how to shower him. We had grab bars in the shower and a shower chair, but it seemed Mark spent most of the time in the shower yelling at me, which of course I couldn't understand what the problem was due to his aphasia. Clearly, I was not doing things in the proper way and he was not happy.

Mark was also waking up two-to-three times during the night to go to the bathroom. I would have to get up with him, help him out of the bed, into his wheelchair and get him down the hall to the handicapped bathroom. It was hard adjusting to not getting a full night's sleep. I had that zombie feeling you get as a new mother who is up all night with your baby. Total exhaustion was setting in.

Thankfully, Mark was capable of going to the bathroom on his own. That had been a serious concern for me, and I was very relieved that he did not need assistance with toileting.

Monday through Friday, Mark went to an outpatient neuro rehab for four hours a day, which was a huge relief. The rehab provided transportation too, which was a big help.

I think it's important to point out here for myself and for others who are in similar situations, that the role of caregiver has been *added* on to our many other roles…

Business Owner.
Mom.
Head of the Household.
Head of Home Maintenance.
Chef.
Housekeeper.
Laundry.
Dealing with yellow jacket infestations (yeah, that actually happened).

It's beyond overwhelming.

I joined Stroke Caregiver Support groups on Facebook to try to pick up some tips on how to balance everything, and make everyone happy. By the way, it's impossible to make everyone happy. It was good to read what others shared and that they were having the same feelings. I realized I wasn't alone and I wasn't a bad person for some of the thoughts that crossed my mind.

I shared a story one day in the group, which had them all "liking it"! It was right after Mark had returned home and I was trying to figure the whole caregiver role out. I am very social and not being able to leave my house even for one day felt like torture to me. One day, Chris was home and I had to run to Walgreens to pick up prescriptions for Mark. It felt so good to be out of my house and in my car alone. Normally, if I were running to Walgreens, I would not be happy to see five cars in front of me, but on this day, it was a beautiful sight. As I sat in my car waiting, I posted this on the caregiver site…

"When you are secretly excited that there are five cars ahead of you at Walgreens because it means you get a longer reprieve from caregiving."

Caregiver humor!
If you're a caregiver you get this with every fiber of your being.

The support group can be helpful, but I had to limit the time I spent on it. Honestly, there were a lot of negative posts and some of the stories were very sad. Some were having serious financial struggles, or had young kids to care for along with their husband. Others were in poor health themselves having to care for a disabled spouse with no help.

I thought to myself, *Suck it up, buttercup – it could be a lot worse.*

YES, it could be worse, but *this* was bad, and in trying to do everything on my own, and believing that it wasn't as bad as what other people were dealing with, I started heading for a breakdown. Thankfully, my friend Karyl, who is a straight shooter said, "Girlfriend, you're not okay. You need to get some help for Mark – and for You." We all need those friends in our lives who tell it like they see it. She was 100% correct.

I immediately reached out to another friend, Lynne, who told me she was using a private caregiver for her mother and loved her. Enter Tiffany the caregiver, or as I called her "my fairy godmother." I hired Tiffany to come three days a week to shower Mark, she was typically there three-to-four hours. When I told Mark I was hiring someone to shower him, he was not happy. In fact, we both cried, but I said to him, I can't do it anymore and you yell at me. Tiffany's first day arrived and they got along great. Showering was easy – she knew what she was doing!

I breathed a huge sigh of relief. I no longer had the dread of shower time hanging over my head, and I was able to spend more time at my office getting work done. Tiffany would take care of things around the house, like fold laundry, clean the kitchen, mop the floors. Seriously, we all fell in love with her.

I had also added a meal delivery service, Front Porch (again thanks to Lynne for the recommendation) so I didn't need to think about cooking during the week. Things were definitely falling into place and I was feeling some relief.

In November 2023, I decided I needed to take a little time for myself. I hadn't seen my mom in over a year, and she was unable to travel due to her husband's ongoing health issues. Chris said he would be fine to care for Mark, plus he had Tiffany for backup, so I scheduled a long weekend trip to Mississippi. It was wonderful to get away, see my family and sleep through the night. For the first time in almost a year, I felt like ME again. I didn't realize how stressed and exhausted I was until I stepped away from my caregiver life for a few days. It was a great way to recharge and I realized it was something I needed to do on a regular basis.

In this caregiving world, I've learned not to get too comfortable because without a doubt things will change. Unfortunately, about six months into our new arrangement, Tiffany had to leave due to personal reasons. We were all sad to lose her, and knew it would be impossible to replace her.

I had leads on a couple of caregivers, but when they no-show an interview, that's a pretty clear sign they're not going to be a good fit. I spoke with several of the Home Care agencies, but they were priced higher than what we could afford, and some couldn't staff the hours we needed.

I was feeling a bit distraught, when an idea occurred to me. I called Chris into my home office and asked him if he felt like he could shower Mark and take over Tiffany's caregiving duties. He said yes, and then I told him, I'm going to pay you to do this. It's only fair. Chris works evenings, so he had to adjust his work schedule to make this work. I made him promise me that if this ever becomes too much for him, to please let me know. I don't want his life to be consumed as his father's caregiver. He just looked at me and said, "Mom, I want to take care of dad." *Have I mentioned that my son is an angel?*

The next day, I arrived home from work, opened the door from the garage into the kitchen and Chris ran toward me, super happy, with an enormous smile on his face and said to me excitedly, "Mom, I gave dad a shower!" My response, "Did he yell at you?" Chris, still smiling, responded with, "Yes, but we figured it out together."

In that moment I clearly understood something very important. This may be a "men versus women" thing, or perhaps just personality type, but Chris does NOT take it personally when Mark gets upset and yells. I do.

I started watching Chris, and if Mark became angry because Chris didn't understand something, Chris would calmly say, "I see" or "Alrighty then," and just walk away. The situation was immediately diffused. Genius.

I am now doing my best to adopt Chris' ways. I call it "What Would Chris Do?" I think I may need a tattoo as a constant reminder!

What I've learned on this caregiving journey, is that it's important to surround yourself with a team, if possible. My current team includes: Chris, a lovely lady named Rebecca who comes on Fridays to help Mark, Abby when she's home from college, my meal delivery service, and a house cleaning service I just hired.

I've realized that I have to protect my health and energy, so I can continue to work and grow my business, while also making sure that Mark is well cared for. I'm not in a position where I can retire any time soon, plus I love my job. It's my passion and truly brings me great joy.

I have noticed, and have been guilty of doing this myself, but people seem to always want to tell caregivers what they *should* be doing. They say things like, "You need to exercise," and "Keep up with your doctor appointments," or "You know the caregiver is more likely to die first." *Okay, we don't need to hear all this. We've heard it over and over and we read it on Google too.*

Instead, let's give resources that may make things easier for the caregiver, for example:

- Use a meal delivery service. The one I use is called Front Porch. They're fresh meals delivered once a week. You simply microwave or heat them in the oven at 350 degrees for 25 minutes. Add a salad and you have a great meal.
- Grocery delivery service. Most of the grocery stores have their own services, or you can use InstaCart.

Or place your order and pickup at your designated time, I've done this at Walmart.

- UberEats every now and then can be worth it or order a pizza. Chris and Mark love pizza and they usually order one on Sundays.
- Pharmacy delivery. I know Walgreens has this service, but check with your local pharmacy.
- If you are not retirement age, like Mark, and disabled, there's a good chance you will qualify for Social Security Disability. It can be difficult to get on your own. I've heard horror stories of people waiting for two years to be approved. The case manager at one of the rehabs told me about a great resource that helps get you approved fast. It's www.allsup.com. They were able to get Mark approved in three months. We first had to wait until he was three months post-stroke to apply. They were very easy to work with, and the extra income has been a big help in offsetting some of the caregiving costs.
- Add a caregiver, even if it's just for a couple of hours.
- Ask family members if they can help.
- If at all possible, try to get away for a night. It's amazing how recharged you will feel having a little time away.
- Create "me time" for yourself. That could be a massage, manicure, reading a book, taking a bath, watching a favorite TV show, etc.
- Don't compare your caregiving situation to others. They may have more challenging circumstances,

but being a caregiver is HARD period. *Never discount your feelings, they are valid and real.*

Caregiving is the hardest job in the world, and there are many people in this role who are hurting and feel invisible. Some caregivers are depressed and feel that their lives are over. If you are constantly feeling this way, please contact your physician. There are medications that can help if needed.

I have always been very anti-med, but I was having difficulty sleeping and experiencing occasional bouts of overwhelming anxiety, brought on when Mark was having a particularly hard day. I have what I refer to as my "happy pill," which is a very low dose of clonazepam. I take only when needed and it does a wonderful job of taking the edge off and calming me down. I'm thankful for that.

*   *   *   *   *

There are also many caregivers who mention that friends have stopped coming to see their loved one. This is heartbreaking.

One of Mark's best friends, Kevin, came to every hospital and rehab he was in, and texted me regularly for updates on how he was doing. Kevin had his own health issues, and had bypass surgery in November 2022, the month before Mark's strokes. He was a wonderful cheerleader for Mark, and when he'd visit I'd leave the room to give them time to catch up. On his last visit he brought Mark a T-shirt that said, "Never Give Up." We were devastated to learn that not long after this, Kevin had a massive heart attack and died. He was only 55.

Telling Mark about Kevin's death was one of the hardest things I've ever had to do. He was devastated. I know without a doubt, if Kevin were still alive he would continue to visit Mark regularly.

I know it's difficult to see a friend become disabled. It's sad to realize that they may not be able to communicate with you in the way they once did. Or maybe they have a progressive disease like Alzheimer's. I will share this with you though… *it is important for you to visit your friend, for your friend's sake.*

Mark has two long-time friends who visit on occasion. He is so excited in the days leading up to their visit, and even though he can't say much, he smiles and nods as they reminisce about past shenanigans. I can tell that these visits help him to feel a sense of normalcy.

CHAPTER 9

Creating and Maintaining a Positive Environment

I am naturally a glass full, happy, and positive person, although my limits have been tested through this journey. Staying positive is important for the entire family as the long road to recovery begins. Incredible results can come from rehab, but if the patient doesn't have the mindset and the will to get better, they won't. Stroke rehab is painful and difficult.

Mark is a hard worker and a fighter. His mom, Cookie, was a single mom raising four kids on her own in the 1960's. Mark is the youngest, and Cookie left his abusive father when he was only three years old. They struggled financially and moved around a lot to stay ahead of the bill collectors. Always a loving and close family, they moved to Arizona at one point to live with family, and then back to the Fort Worth area when Mark was in high school.

Mark showed signs of being a go-getter from the time he was still a young child. I've always loved this story he told me. I think he was around ten years old, and he would stop every day at a small, local store at the same time the bread delivery truck was arriving. He'd help put the bread from the truck onto the shelves. I think the store owner paid him something, but what I always remember from this story is that Mark's mom couldn't afford to buy a bike for him. One day, close to Christmas, Mark stopped at the store to help put the bread on the shelves. The store owner and the delivery driver had a surprise for him…a brand new bike!

He first told me this story when we were dating, and I burst into tears. I always intended to write the story down, but never did until now.

Throughout life, Mark has battled with severe depression. As has happened to many people, he was laid off from a job he had been at for seventeen years. He loved where he worked and fully believed he would retire there. Losing this job affected him deeply, he took it personally. Not long before his stroke we were talking about it, and I asked him if he had ever gotten over it. He said, "No."

Knowing Mark as well as I do, I was concerned about his tendency toward negativity and his struggles with depression. I knew he had the strong will and work ethic needed in the battle for recovery. As a family, I had no doubt that we would do everything possible to help him to remain positive and fighting even on his darkest days.

One of the biggest motivators for Mark to work hard in rehab was to come home and be with our dogs. He loves all animals, especially our two elderly dogs, Teddy (Yorkshire Terrier) and Dexter (Yorkie/Shih Tzu mix), and our golden retriever puppy, Sadie. I'm pretty sure that Sadie may be the love of his life!

In February 2022, Abby was home from college and she and I were talking about how much we loved golden retrievers. I had a golden, Champ, when I was a child, and we had an incredible golden, Sage, when the kids were little. Sadly, he died right before his ninth birthday from cancer. We were all completely devastated by the loss of such a wonderful dog.

Abby found a lady in Wichita Falls whose golden retriever had just had a litter of puppies in January. She messaged back and forth with the lady, and we told her we wanted a female puppy. We made all of the arrangements, and then we went to tell Mark. He was less than thrilled and told us NO!

Of course, as you may know by now, the word "no" doesn't always register with me.

The date came when we could go visit the puppies, now six weeks old, and pick out the one we wanted. I told Mark, and he said "no," and he kept saying "no" the entire two-hour drive to Wichita Falls. We walked into the lady's house and were greeted by a dozen, bouncing, wiggling, energetic six-week-old golden retriever puppies.

Let me say right now, I am going to be extremely disappointed if this is not what heaven looks like!

Chris laid on the floor and was immediately covered in puppies. Abby scooped up a puppy and cuddled it in her arms, and Mark stood there smiling ear to ear, while the chubbiest male puppy begged for his attention…which he got!

We decided on a little girl who was wearing a pink collar because pink was my grandmother's favorite color. The puppies had been born on January 28th, but when I told the lady why I picked the puppy with the pink collar, she got a funny look on her face. She said she wasn't sharing this information with everyone, but the puppy with the pink collar was actually the first and only puppy born on January 27th. That's our anniversary! I believe in signs and this was a sign that could not be ignored. She was definitely meant to be our puppy.

We had to wait another two weeks to pick her up, as she had to be eight weeks old. Mark made some feeble attempts to say "no," but it was obvious he was already smitten with her. The day finally came to bring Sadie home, and who did she immediately attach herself to? Mark, of course.

From the day she came home, she shadowed Mark and he absolutely loved every second of it. We taught her to ring a bell that hung on the back door to let us know when she needed to go outside. She took to ringing the bell whenever she needed anything. I teasingly told Mark that he was her butler.

I'm sure Sadie was very confused when her best friend and constant companion suddenly disappeared on Christmas Day. Chris did a great job stepping in and caring for her, but still she missed her daddy.

While Mark was still in the hospital, I would show him pictures and videos of Sadie. That would always get a smile out of him. When he moved to the live-in rehabilitation center, I ordered a stuffed golden retriever puppy for him. While he was in therapy, I decorated his room with the goal of making it feel a bit like home. My friend Kathy had sent him a cozy blanket covered in scripture. I put that on his bed, added framed pictures of our family at Disney World, a picture of Mark with his mom, and a picture of Sadie. Lastly, I put the stuffed puppy on his pillow. His eyes lit up when he saw it. I found out later that he slept every night with that stuffed puppy. When he finally returned home he set it on his night stand, where it remains today. Sadie occasionally takes an interest in it, but Mark is quick to tell her, "No."

Forty-five days after his stroke, Mark had a doctor's appointment with his primary care physician whose office happens to be directly across from our neighborhood. The rehab would transport Mark to the appointment. I asked if they could possibly come a little early, so Mark could have a brief reunion with Sadie. They were kind enough to say yes. On a cold, rainy day Mark and Sadie were reunited. I made a TikTok video of their reunion. I'm so happy to have documented this beautiful moment.

The rehab allowed us to bring Sadie there to visit, but she had to remain outdoors. Chris and I brought her twice. It was a 45-minute to one-hour drive to the rehab, depending on traffic, and Sadie is not the best car traveler. Let's just say there is lots of panting, drooling, and shedding. Mark enjoyed spending time with her, and we even were allowed to take her to an outdoor party where other rehab patients had gathered. It was incredible how she instinctively knew who wanted to pet her and who didn't. She was only a little over a year old at the time, which for a golden retriever is still in the hyper puppy years. Amazingly, she was calm and quiet.

Sadie has been Mark's constant companion since he returned home in July. She is not officially trained as a therapy dog, but has stepped into that role (self-trained!). When he gets up to go to the bathroom, she follows him and lays outside the bathroom door waiting for him. She lays at his feet while he watches TV, and if we would allow her, she'd sleep in the bed on top of him.

I have several family members and friends who have said Sadie is an Angel sent to our family to help us through this difficult time. God knew what was coming, so maybe he did send her. I'm just glad she's part of our family.

While Mark was living at the rehab, I only visited on weekends. He was in therapy all day, and after dinner and a shower, there wasn't much time to visit. Not to mention, it was a long drive to make every day and still maintain my work schedule. I didn't want him to feel forgotten, so I made sure to call every day to talk to him. I couldn't understand what he was saying, but I could tell by his tone that he was happy I had called.

I noticed that he loved receiving cards, so I posted on Facebook that Get Well cards made Mark happy. The cards flooded in! I would bring a stack every time I visited and we would open them together. He loved seeing who the card was from, and he always seemed a bit amazed that so many people were thinking of him. I asked the rehab if I could tape the cards on his wall, and they said yes. Unfortunately, the tape wasn't strong enough to stick them to the wall and they kept falling off. My friend Karyl came up with a solution. She found a hanger for the door with clips to attach the cards to. I also found a way to string cards up over his bed, and of course there were cards on his bureau and his night stand.

I wanted him to feel surrounded by the healing love of our family and friends, and he was.

All of the therapists at the hospital and rehabs we encountered were kind and professional, but there was one who stood out in a big way.

Mark's longest stay was at Pate, the live-in rehab. He was there from late January until mid-July. During that time his Physical Therapist was an incredible young woman named Sara. She was tough, which Mark needed and responded to. He arrived in a wheelchair, unable to transfer in and out of it on his own. He left, walking with the use of a cane. Mark adored and respected Sara, as did our entire family. She would send me videos of Mark as he learned to walk again, which I would share with our family and on social media. It helped me to see how Mark was progressing in therapy, since I wasn't able to be there every day. I'm so thankful that Sara was a part of Mark's recovery journey.

The live-in rehab had two houses. One for people who needed a lot of care, and another that was basically set up like an assisted living. It had a private apartment with a kitchenette and a small patio. There was a dining room where everyone gathered for meals, and care staff to manage medications and help with showers, and other care needs. Mark started in the first house, and was there for most of his stay. He was so excited when he finally got word that he was moving to the other house. His move was almost put on hold when he had a fall in the bathroom the night before he was to move. Luckily, he only had a couple of bruises, and was still able to move the next day.

I was there to move all of his belongings to the new house, and get him settled in. We saw several familiar faces from the first house. One of the men greeted Mark and welcomed him with a bag of chocolates. I learned much later that this was actually contraband, as they were supposed to be on healthy diets. Obviously, most were there because they'd had strokes.

By this time, I had started to bring Mark home on Saturdays for the day. He loved being home and with Sadie. One day after a visit, I was driving him back to rehab when he insisted that I stop at the grocery store. I couldn't understand what he wanted, but I stopped. I got his wheelchair out, helped him into it, and he directed me where to go. I pushed him through the store, until he found what he wanted. The candy aisle? Yep, and he picked out the biggest bag of chocolates I've ever seen. I didn't want him to eat all of this candy, and I couldn't understand why he wanted such a large bag, but he was adamant so I gave in and bought the candy.

We got back to the rehab and he asked me to open the bag, and that's when I learned what he was up to. He wasn't going to eat the candy, he wanted to *give* candy to the new people who had moved to the house, and welcome them just like the man had done for him.

He was paying it forward.

CHAPTER 10

Modifying Your Home

For the first two months after Mark's strokes I clung to the hope that he would recover 100%. I read stories of other people who'd had similar strokes and recovered fully. However, as time went by, I realized the stroke had caused significant injuries to his brain and that he would likely be disabled to some extent.

During a meeting in March at his rehab, the Occupational Therapist mentioned that she could schedule a visit to our home, bring Mark with her and make recommendations for modifications. At that time, the rehab had given Mark an approximate discharge date in May. I knew it would take time to make the needed changes to our home, so I asked her to come as soon as possible. We scheduled the visit for the end of March.

Mark had not been home since leaving abruptly for the ER on Christmas Day, and I was excited to see him come through the front door. Around the time they were scheduled to arrive, I received a call from the therapist, she said, "I think we are at the wrong house. Mark says this isn't his house?" I verified the address with her as I walked to the front of the house. Through the front window I saw the rehab van in my driveway, but Mark continued to tell her she was at the wrong house. I walked out to the van, and then it dawned on me why he was confused.

In early November, we had completed repairs to the front of our house caused by a car backing into it. Mark had sold a couple of tables to an older woman on Facebook Marketplace. She came to pick them up in her van, and as she backed the van up our driveway she accidentally confused the gas and the brake. She floored it, hitting Mark, who was thankfully thrown out of the way and then slammed her van into the brick between the garage doors. After a prolonged fight with insurance, the repairs to the house had been completed in November. The entire garage had been rebuilt and new garage doors installed. We had changed the style of the doors and that's what had thrown Mark off. This is also when I realized he had no memories from about late October prior to the stroke. It's like they've just been completely erased.

Once I explained to Mark that the repairs had been made, he settled down and was ready to come into the house. The Occupational Therapist had also brought another therapist with her, and it's a good thing she did. Just getting Mark's wheelchair over the threshold of the front door was a challenge.

Mark was of course elated to be home, and Sadie gave him a very warm welcome! We began going through the house with Mark and the therapists checking to see what modifications would need to be done...

- Front door needed a ramp
- None of the doorways to the bathrooms were wide enough for wheelchair access
- Shower modification and grab bars needed in shower and by toilet
- Bed was too low, and because it's a Sleep Number bed, a pole would need to be installed next to the bed
- Kitchen table was too high for the wheelchair
- And the list went on and on.

To say I was overwhelmed was an understatement.

I wanted our home functional for Mark, but I also cared about the aesthetic of our home. Some of the suggestions, like "remove the doors to the bathroom cabinets to give him access to the sink" made me cringe inside. We remodeled our master bathroom several years ago, and it's my favorite place in the house, because it has a relaxing, spa feel. The therapist's suggestion was to remove the glass around the shower and rig a shower curtain around it. No way was that going to happen! I would find a better way to create a safe environment for Mark, without destroying our house.

We moved to Dallas in 1997. Chris was ten months old, and it was important to me that we find a house with a master bedroom and another bedroom downstairs. I wanted my baby close to me and on the same floor. Not an easy thing to find in the late-90's, when most of the homes were built with all bedrooms upstairs. One weekend, we were driving around and found a brand new neighborhood. There was a house in the process of being built, and it was EXACTLY what we were looking for – master bedroom and another bedroom plus full bathroom downstairs. We bought it!

I will never forget Mark saying, *"When we're old and can't go up the stairs we will just live downstairs."* Those prophetic words came back to me 27 years later (except I don't consider us old yet).

I decided that we would leave the master bathroom alone, and convert the full bathroom downstairs into an accessible bathroom for Mark. My friend Aricia Blasko is not only a well-known realtor in our area, but she also has an excellent reputation for remodeling bathrooms and kitchens. I called her and we scheduled a time to meet. I loved her idea to remove a hallway closet so we could widen the bathroom door, remove the bathtub and build a huge open shower. Aricia brought her carpenter over, and he offered to build a handicap accessible cabinet for the sink. I know he gave me a deep discount too, which I greatly appreciated. They were able to remove the quartz from on top of the existing cabinet and reuse it, which helped save money.

Aricia then told me that she had talked to several of my neighbors and friends, and they all wanted to help. The men did some of the work, like putting in grab bars, a new light fixture and faucet. Others purchased paint and helped chipped in to pay for items needed. My mother and stepfather loaned me the money to pay the contractors for the remodel. I am crying as I write this and remembering the generosity of our family, friends, and neighbors.

As the bathroom remodel began, I started my search for the best items to purchase for modifying our home. Most could be found on Amazon of course. I feel certain that the delivery driver was quietly cursing me as he delivered the insanely heavy ramps for my front and back doors. I have no idea how much they weigh, but they work perfectly! I ordered grab bars, a shower chair and other items suggested by the Occupational Therapist.

I did end up returning several items once I had Mark home and realized we could manage without them. One was the pole for the bedroom. It actually looked a bit like a stripper pole. The therapist was concerned Mark wouldn't have the strength to get out of our bed without the pole. We have a Sleep Number bed, which was lower than what was recommended, and we couldn't attach any kind of rail to the mattress. It ended up being a non-issue. I could help Mark by holding his hand as he used me for support. Now that he's stronger he can sit up on his own and use his wheelchair as support to get up on his own.

The bathroom was completed in early-May. Now, with a fully accessible bathroom I was able to start bringing Mark home on Saturdays. This gave us a great opportunity to work through some obstacles. My sister-in-law Dianne was with me the first time we brought Mark home for the day. We were struggling trying to push Mark's wheelchair up the ramp and into the house. One of my neighbors saw us, and ran over to assist. We realized we needed to BACK his wheelchair up the ramp. That made it much easier! We also discovered that his wheelchair was a perfect fit for the island in the kitchen. The height was perfect and that has now become his spot for meals.

Chris and I had already moved throw rugs and furniture to allow Mark access. We made a few additional adjustments once he was in the home, to give him more room to get around in his wheelchair.

One thing I became keenly aware of when I started bringing Mark home for visits, was that my car was not the best fit for either of us. I had a seven-year-old Lincoln MKX, which is a good sized SUV. I loved that car, and not just because it was paid off. The problem was, it was a struggle for Mark to get in it, plus it was almost impossible for me to put his wheelchair in the back. I'm short (5'2") and admittedly not physically very strong. I had to take off most of the attachments to his wheelchair, so I could fold it and then using all of my strength, hoist it up and into the back of my SUV. It was not a pretty sight, and I was afraid of injuring my back.

I knew I needed to buy a minivan, but I didn't want to.

One, because of the expense of a new car and two, it was a minivan. We had minivans when the kids were little and honestly, I did love the convenience they offered, but at 59 years old, I was not excited about the prospect of becoming a minivan driver.

Practicality, and the fear of a back injury won out. I began the search for a minivan. I decided on the Chrysler Pacifica, because the seats easily fold flat, perfect for a wheelchair. I found one with all the extras – sunroof, sport package, etc., that had been purchased and returned. I guess the people decided they weren't minivan drivers. It had less than 1,000 miles on it, and I was able to negotiate a good deal. At least, I think it was a good deal – buying a car is a torturous experience.

As I turned over the keys to my Lincoln, I may have shed a tear or two. I drove off in my very large minivan, headed home and "docked" it in my garage. It felt more like a ship than a car! As I got out of it, I laughed at how HUGE it was. Seriously, there is hardly any space to walk around this beast. I immediately christened her "Large Marge."

I have posted about Large Marge on social media, and it always amuses me that people never refer to her as my van, they all call her Large Marge. She has gained quite the following!

I will admit this publicly now…I love Large Marge. It's easy for Mark to get in and out and I can pick up his wheelchair, without folding it or taking off any attachments, and easily plop it in the back of the van.

* * * * *

No one ever imagines that a catastrophic illness or accident will happen to their family. I know I never gave it much thought, and if I did, I'm sure I didn't get past thinking of the emotional side of it, or the medical debt.

The financial hit on a family goes way beyond just hospital bills. There is the ripple effect of ongoing medical care, lost income for the injured person, loss of wages for the primary caregiver, expensive modifications needed for the home, caregivers, expense of an accessible vehicle, and the list goes on.

I am aware of how blessed we are to be surrounded by family and friends who helped us during this dark time. I look back on it now and I am in awe of how everyone came together to help my family. Their kindness and generosity will never be forgotten.

CHAPTER 11

Grieving Someone Who is Still Alive

This has been the hardest chapter for me to write; in fact, I put off writing it as long as I could.

The idea of grieving someone who is still alive may sound odd, but when someone you love has suffered a catastrophic illness or accident that has changed them physically, mentally, or both, you do grieve the person they were.

I've experienced the loss of people I love – my dad, my grandparents, aunts, uncles, and my best friend Beth from childhood. You expect to feel grief when someone you love dies, but what surprised me were the waves of grief I felt for Mark in the months following his strokes and still feel at times.

Most of us are probably familiar with Elisabeth Kübler-Ross' five stages of grief – denial, anger, bargaining, depression, and acceptance. I have gone through all of these phases since Mark's strokes.

Even though Mark is still here, and he is still who he always was, there are things about him that I miss and grieve. There are moments of crushing sadness for our pre-stroke lives. I remember being caught off guard when the initial waves of grief hit me, but once I acknowledged what I was feeling, I decided that as these thoughts occurred to me, I would write them in a journal. I found it to be very cathartic.

These are some of the many things I miss…

I miss the way Mark walked. He's a big guy, and he always walked with great purpose and strength. He was always the rock who took care of all the things that needed tending to around the house. I can envision him on a ladder fixing things, and believe me that man loves his ladders. I think there are at least five in the garage. I grieve this part of him, because I know it's gone forever..

I miss the sound of his voice, and I call his voicemail every now and then just to hear it. The stroke has affected his speech and even though he can talk some, it's not like before. Although, we do still pray that he will continue to improve.

I miss the things he did that annoyed me. When we were watching TV, Mark always knew the actors and what show they were in thirty years ago. He would always pause what we were watching to share this information with me. I would get annoyed, and tell him to just put the show back on. I've since apologized to him for being so mean. He still knows all of the actors, but now I have to try to figure out who they are and their names, because he can't verbalize it.

I miss the fact that he can no longer drive. He loved to drive, and did the majority of the driving when we were together. To be honest, he was one of those aggressive Dallas drivers, going way too fast and weaving in and out of traffic. My eyes were closed much of the time, as I yelled slow down! Now, I'm the sole driver, and I don't like it.

I miss him being there for Chris and Abby the way he was. He was the dad that would do absolutely anything for his kids. When Abby was going to school in Oklahoma City, he drove her back after a weekend at home. It's a three-hour drive from our house, and about ten minutes from her dorm, she remembered that she'd forgotten her school ID. He wasn't happy, but he drove the three hours back to Oklahoma City the next day to give her the ID and then three hours back home.

I miss his cooking. He made the most amazing meatballs stuffed with cheese. The last time he cooked them was Christmas Eve, the day before his stroke.

I miss going on trips together, especially Disney World with the kids. I don't know if this will ever be possible again, but it certainly won't look the way it used to.

In addition to all of the things I miss about Mark, I'm angry that the stroke happened on Christmas Day. We love Christmas, but unfortunately, we will always remember what happened on Christmas Day 2022.

There were many times in the first year when intense feelings of sadness or anger would overcome me. These feelings still pop up on occasion, but not as intense as they were

I think people don't like to talk about anger, especially women, but it is a human emotion and one that is okay to express and get out of your system. Of course, I'm not saying stomp around angrily, yelling at the clerks at the grocery store. That would be unhealthy anger.

It's also important that we remember not to compare our situation to others. This again may be something more women are prone to do. There were many times when I would think to myself, *Why did this happen to us?* Only to have the next thought be, *Well, it could be worse. At least the kids are young adults and not toddlers.* True, but this situation does suck. And it's okay to feel sad for yourself, to feel angry at God, to scream like a maniac in your car or garage. I have experienced all of these. Quite honestly, I think I would've exploded or had a mental breakdown if I hadn't gotten these feelings out.

Mark's rehab was a 45-minute drive from our house. There were many days when I'd leave the rehab after a visit, especially if Mark was having a bad day, and literally scream in my car. Sometimes I'd have conversations with God, asking him why this had happened or praying for the strength to get through it.

I am very close to my brother and his wife, and felt comfortable sharing my innermost thoughts with them. They were there for all of my ups and downs as I processed each new challenge that seemed to present itself on a daily basis. Also, I have a handful of ride-or-die friends. Those friends who will be at your house at midnight with a bottle of wine if you need them. I knew I could tell them anything without fear of judgment.

It's part of grief to go through this anger stage, and I think we get in trouble if we don't have a release for the anger, or if we attempt to deny how we are feeling.

Feelings of sadness are expected when you are navigating your way through a loved one's catastrophic illness. I felt extreme sadness that this would happen on Christmas Day, and that my kids were only 26 and 19. I also thought about how hard it was for me not to have my dad walk me down the aisle when I got married. I don't want that for my daughter. I want her dad to be able to be there to give her away, even if he's in a wheelchair or using a cane to walk her down the aisle.

Sadness is absolutely a normal emotion to feel, but if you find yourself feeling hopeless and depressed, *please seek help.* Therapy and medication can be life savers.

For me, the acceptance stage kind of snuck up on me. One day, I realized our lives are forever changed. It's not the life we had planned for, and that is sad. However, Mark is still here with us, and that is a miracle. We are still creating happy, joyful memories together.

Will there be moments of anger and sadness? Of course, but we will process through them and continue to move forward.

CHAPTER 12

The Roller Coaster Continues

As Christmas 2023 approached, and the one year anniversary of Mark's stroke, I was torn about decorating the house. Ultimately, the kids and I decided that there was a lot to celebrate and decorated the house. Our sweet neighbor Sole prepared a feast and shared it with us for Christmas dinner. We ate earlier in the day, so when 7:00 p.m. rolled around, we weren't in the kitchen reliving memories of last year.

As 2024 approached, I was honestly happy to bid 2023 farewell. I was excited about the new year, I'd even come up with a new word for the year, which has since been forgotten, and had thoughts of creating a vision board. I spent all of New Year's Day packing away our Christmas decorations. I usually wait until the sixth, but I wanted my house back to normal. I had new projects ready to get started on for work, plus I was ready to commit time to writing this book. I was raring to go in the new year!

January 2nd, Mark went to rehab as normal. We had dinner, he watched TV, all was normal except he was feeling tired and wanted to go to bed a little earlier.

Around 1:00 a.m., he woke up and needed to go to the bathroom, so I helped him down the hall. I jumped back in bed, which is normal, and listened for him. He was taking a long time, so I went to check on him. He said he had a stomach ache. Finally, I heard the bathroom door open and he made it halfway down the hall and stopped. He looked at me, and I knew he was about to vomit. I got him back to the bathroom and he started throwing up. By then, it was about 2:00 a.m. and I called Chris on my phone. He was asleep upstairs, and asked him to come help me. It's a lot to care for someone who is in a wheelchair and is sick with a stomach virus – everything was coming out of both ends.

Not to be too graphic, but I believe what he had was viral because the smell was overwhelming. I was trying to help and clean up, but was gagging and close to vomiting. Chris looked at me and said, "Mom, I've got this." God bless him, he cleaned everything up. Of course, these types of viruses come in waves, so he'd be okay for an hour and then it would start up again.

In our marriage, I can only recall Mark throwing up once, maybe twice. He's one of those people who rarely even had a cold. I wasn't too concerned until about 5:00 a.m. He had thrown up again, but then had settled into his recliner and fallen asleep. I called my sister-in-law Dianne because I knew they'd be up early and asked her if I should call 911. I felt like I might be overreacting a bit, and she said check him for fever, but if he's sleeping just let him rest. Which absolutely made sense, since he was fever free.

I laid on the couch and watched over him for the next couple of hours. At 7:00 a.m., he woke up and wanted to go to the bathroom. I positioned his wheelchair for him, and he started trying to transfer from his recliner. He made a joke like he was falling, which is one of his usual pranks (remember, he's always been a practical joker). On maybe the fourth time trying to get up, he fell back into his recliner, leaning to the left and started to have a seizure.

I had never seen a seizure, and I would wish that on no one. I screamed for Chris, who was on the couch in the other room. I was doing my best not to panic, but realized I was holding my phone and telling Chris to call 911. I quickly gathered my wits, and called 911. Chris and I were standing close to the recliner, making sure Mark didn't fall out as he continued to have the seizure. I remember trying to keep my voice calm and tell the operator what was happening. I know it probably took five minutes for them to get there, but it felt like an eternity.

At some point the intense seizure stopped, and I noticed that Mark's eyes were gazing off to the right, unblinking and he was making very odd, irregular breathing sounds. I started to panic, and asked the operator if they were almost here. I was completely unnerved that he wasn't blinking his eyes and said to the operator I think he's dying. At this point, the operator asked me to start counting every time he took a breath. As I type this, I realize he likely did that to keep me from going into a panic attack and staying present in the moment with a task.

We finally heard the sirens approaching and I told Chris to go open the front door. After that it's a bit of a blur. I remember lots of firemen coming in, one asked me about medications, so I took him to the kitchen where I had created a list and put it on the refrigerator. On the list, I had all of Mark's meds, his doctors, diagnosis, etc. One of the firemen asked if I had a preference for the hospital –yes, he's a stroke survivor, please take him to Medical City Lewisville. I wanted to be sure Mark had access to neurologists familiar with strokes.

I sort of remember them loading him on the gurney – he was completely unresponsive. Chris and I hugged tightly in the kitchen and all I could think was, *This is really bad.*

I threw on some clothes, brushed my teeth and put a hat on. The day before, I was drying my hair when suddenly my hair started smoking. My very old hair dryer had almost caught my hair on fire, and I had a singe mark across the side of my hair. I had an appointment to fix it that day, which of course I had to cancel. Oh well, it was winter and I had borrowed a cute hat from Abby.

The ambulance was in my driveway for what felt like an eternity. I didn't know if that was good or bad. My next door neighbor texted and said they were praying for Mark. As soon as the ambulance pulled out, I got in my car to follow them to the ER, calling my brother and mom to let them know what was going on.

The ER was packed. It was January, so of course there were lots of illnesses going around. Mark was still pretty out of it, and the nurses were trying to figure out his baseline. The normal questions are always, what's your name and when is your date of birth. I explained to them that he is a stroke survivor with severe aphasia and is unable to answer those questions.

I felt some relief when he opened his eyes, but he wasn't really focusing, and he started this non-stop babble like he was talking to someone. The nurses took his temp and he had a fever of 104.3!

We were in the ER until around 4:00 p.m., when they finally had a room available for him. He was still very out of it. They had started him on seizure medications. It's not uncommon to develop a seizure disorder after having a stroke. They weren't sure if the seizure was from that or due to being dehydrated and having such a high fever. It was another awful long day and night. By the next morning he was doing much better.

Tiffany, our wonderful caregiver, came to sit with him so I could run home and take a shower. Abby was at her boyfriend's house and asked if I could stop by and pick her up on the way to the hospital. She was worried and wanted to see Mark.

I mentioned previously that I had traded in my beloved SUV for a minivan, Large Marge. I was still a little cranky about driving a minivan, but of course it made life easier getting Mark in and out.

I was enroute to pick up Abby, talking to her through Bluetooth, when I noticed out of the corner of my eye a car moving way too fast out of a parking lot. I tried to move into the left lane and speed up a bit, but he was going too fast, then BANG, he crashed into the right rear of Large Marge. He hit so hard, I felt the right side of the van lift up off the road. I had a momentary thought that it was going to flip, but thankfully it didn't.

Abby said I screamed in fear. It wasn't fear, I was just so freaking pissed off! I will now admit to probably one of my worst mom moments ever. Abby hears the crash, my scream…and then I just hung up the phone. She's freaking out and calls Chris. So now, here are my poor kids, one parent extremely ill in the hospital, and now their mom has been in a wreck and they have no idea if I'm dead or injured.

No one was injured, thankfully, however Marge was severely injured to the tune of $15,000 worth of damage. Yep, not even 7,000 miles on the odometer. That sucks.

The guy who hit me said the sun was in his eyes, which still doesn't really explain flying out of a parking lot into a person who is minding their own business just driving down the road.

I called 911 for the second day in a row. The guy who hit me was worried because he saw the handicapped plates and thought he had hit a handicapped person. No, I assured him. The handicapped person is currently in the hospital.

The police came, the guy admitted fault of course, and another man who had witnessed the wreck gave me his card in case I needed a witness.

Then, I remembered I needed to call my kids! Chris answered on the first ring, with a frazzled, "Mom! Are you okay?" Both kids were very relieved that I was okay, and I asked Chris to come pick me up since my car was undrivable and about to be towed away.

While on the side of the road, the hospital called and asked if I would like for Mark to go to their hospital rehab, once he was feeling better. He would need intense rehab to get back to his baseline after being so ill. As we talked, there were cars whizzing past me, and she said, it sounds like you're on the side of the road. Oh, well that's because I am, and I told her what had just happened. She couldn't believe it. Neither could I!

2024 was not off to a good start.

Chris arrived and we started getting my stuff out of Large Marge and transferring it to his car. The police officer was super nice and was helping. I noticed something under my driver's seat, oh great, it was a bottle of wine in a Christmas bag. I pulled it out and said to her, "Okay, this is wine and it's unopened and I am really going to need it tonight." She laughed!

After calls to insurance, I picked up a rental car and Abby and I made it to the hospital about two hours later than initially planned.

Mark was looking much better and was coherent again. He understood that I had been in a wreck, but was okay.

He spent the next five days in the hospital and then moved to their hospital rehab. Of all the hospitals and rehabs we had been to over the past year, this one was the best. It was on the smaller side, and all of the staff were wonderful. Mark was treated like a king, and he said the food was delicious too. I kind of think he wanted to stay!

January 2024 had more challenges in store. While Mark was still in rehab, Dallas was hit with a winter storm. I felt prepared because we had new pool equipment installed a couple of years prior and based on the fancy app on my phone, freeze protection had been activated. As I snuggled up into a warm blanket to read a book, I had a nagging feeling come over me. I kept thinking, if Mark was here he would go outside and check the pool equipment. I couldn't shake the thought, so

I bundled up, pulled on my boots and trudged out into the cold. The equipment is on the other side of my house, and as I turned the corner, I saw the most shocking sight. Water had been shooting out of the pump and had frozen all over the equipment and on the wall.

I apologize to any of my neighbors who may have been outside at that time, because I yelled every curse word I knew and made up a few new ones too.

A friend who owns a pool company had her husband come by. He performed a temporary fix to get me through it. I finally was able to reach the pool company that services my pool and they came the next day. By this time, my pool had ice formed on top of it. That's not a sight you witness often in Dallas. His advice was to use my shovel to break it up every few hours. I did, and surprisingly it was kind of fun. I released a lot of anger into that ice.

The next challenge to present itself was heartbreaking. Our little yorkie, Teddy, was 15 years old and had been declining for quite a while. We knew it was time to have him put to sleep, but we selfishly could not bring ourselves to make that final decision. Chris and I talked about it and felt like Mark should see Teddy one last time.

Unfortunately, while Mark was still in rehab, Teddy declined further. One morning, Chris was outside with Teddy, who could no longer see or hear well, when he fell into the pool. Chris saw it happen, and got to Teddy immediately. We wrapped him in towels, but noticed that one of his back legs was bent at an awkward angle. He didn't seem to be in pain, thankfully, but we knew the time had come. I called our vet, who was booked up. They gave me the name of another vet, who was available and told us to come in right away. Chris and I held Teddy and told him how much we loved him and what a good boy he was as the injections were given to him. His passing was very peaceful.

I went to the rehab afterwards to tell Mark what had happened. He was sad, but indicated to me that he knew we had made the right decision for Teddy.

Finally the day arrived when Mark's rehab stay came to an end and he returned home to resume normal life again, returning to his regular outpatient neuro rehab.

It took six weeks for poor Large Marge to return from her "rehab." Plus, lots of arguments with insurance.

What I learned from this latest twist in our stroke journey is that Mark's body is compromised. His body is not like it was pre-stroke. Minor illnesses can have extreme effects on him. Chris ended up getting the same stomach virus, but it was mild and only lasted a couple of days.

Life is going to be a rollercoaster ride from now on (*minus any more car accidents, I hope*). Caring for someone with a chronic health condition has many ups and downs.

The biggest struggle, at least for me, is to not let anxiety take over and live in a world of expecting the worst to happen. It's easy to let fear take over, especially after all the challenges thrown at us in January 2024.

What helps me, is to remind myself every day to just stay in the moment and not to overthink the what-if's.

I would be lying if I didn't admit to feelings of PTSD after witnessing Mark's seizure. As bad as seeing him have his strokes, this was so much worse.

It may sound like an overreaction, but if he ever throws up again, I am calling 911!

CHAPTER 13

Releasing Feelings of Guilt

Caregiving and feelings of guilt go hand in hand, you don't find one without the other unfortunately. Most guilt is self-induced and grows as you become increasingly overwhelmed in your situation.

There is an incredible amount of responsibility that comes when you step into the role of caregiver. Mark needed me to care for pretty much his every need – take him to doctor's appointments, manage his medications, help him shower, dress, put on his leg and arm braces, make sure he ate nutritious meals, and on and on. Not to mention, all of the other things I needed to do to keep my business and household running.

When Mark returned home in July, and I became his primary caregiver, I was obsessed with doing everything right.

My goal was to be the best caregiver possible. Quickly, I found myself doubting some of my decisions and listening to that nagging little voice in my head that was telling me I was doing everything wrong.

Mark wasn't exactly easy to care for, and prone to anger and yelling in the beginning. When you're doing your best to help someone and they yell at you, the natural response is to feel anger. He would yell, I would be silently pissed (sometimes not so silent), and then I would remember he has a brain injury, which would result in feelings of guilt because how can I be mad at someone with a brain injury. It was a vicious cycle.

I felt that I was failing Chris and Abby too. Especially Abby. She was always daddy's girl, and he spoiled her rotten. Now that constant support was missing from her life, and I simply didn't have the time or energy to be there as much as she needed. Of course, this led to more feelings of guilt for me.

Around this time, I became completely overwhelmed and close to an emotional breakdown. If you remember, in an earlier chapter I shared about this. My friend Karyl stepped in and told me it was time to bring in help. Her firm, yet kind words were sort of like that get yourself together slap across the face you often see in old movies. It was exactly what I needed to push me out of my downward cycle of guilt and realize that I was not Wonder Woman, and could not handle everything on my own.

Awareness of where the guilt was coming from and providing myself with grace helped a lot in easing those feelings. It's normal to feel anger and resentment at times toward the one you are caring for. Because I was so overwhelmed these feelings were magnified. Once I brought in a caregiver to help Mark with his showers, things started to change.

I also realized that I was giving Mark a pass on his bad behavior, and decided it was time for a new approach. When he would become angry and yell, I would calmly state… "I will not be yelled at," and I would leave the room. Sometimes, I would go in the garage for a minute and rant to myself. When I would return, he was always calm. It didn't take long for him to catch on that his behavior was unacceptable.

Changing my reaction to his behavior made him aware that his yelling would not be tolerated. In turn, this brought more peace to our home, which resulted in releasing some of the guilt I was feeling.

I have found that guilt also creeps in when you have moments of grief over the future you had planned. We had big plans for our future, including lots of travel to Alaska, Italy, Ireland, etc. I wanted to go everywhere and see everything. Mark's dream was to buy an RV and drive all over the country. The kind of travel we planned is not a reality now.

I think about one day fulfilling my travel dreams, but the thought of leaving Mark for an extended period of time and to travel so far away fills me with guilt. I feel badly that he won't get to experience things that I will, and I also worry about him getting sick while I'm gone.

I have gone on short trips to Mississippi to see my family, and have returned feeling energized and refreshed. Chris and Abby are wonderful caregivers, and I trust them to take great care of Mark while I'm gone.

In addition to the self-imposed guilt that caregivers struggle with, there is also the guilt we feel from other people who question or judge decisions we have made. It's easy to say the words, I don't care what others think of me, because they have never spent a day in my shoes, BUT it still gets under your skin, their words embedding into your thoughts.

When Mark became ill with his stomach virus and subsequent seizure in January, he ended up needing to go to rehab to regain his strength. As luck would have it, his discharge date was on Saturday, January 20th. I had a trip planned to Mississippi that weekend to see my brother Craig, who was being crowned King of his Mardi Gras Krewe. This was a big deal, and I was excited to spend time with family and friends, celebrating Craig as he received this honor.

Mark was doing great, and Chris felt confident that he would be fine with the rehab discharge process and getting Mark settled in at home. Abby would be there too, and Mark's caregiver was on standby. I felt pretty good about things, although I told Craig, the moment the plane takes off will be the moment I am sure that I'm coming. I had a few twinges of guilt, but felt good about my decision…until a friend texted and asked, "Are you sure about going on this trip? That's a lot to ask Chris to handle." Whoa, that text threw me into guilt overload!

I finally calmed myself down, and thought about the plans I had made. Chris is a 27-year-old man. He had been helping me with Mark's care for over a year. Just to be sure though, I asked Chris if he felt he could handle things if I went on the trip. He looked at me like I was crazy, and said, "Yes, of course, Mom."

I went on the trip. Chris and Abby did a fantastic job caring for their dad, and I had a wonderful time.

People will always have opinions, and I'm sure this friend was well-intentioned and didn't intend to send me into a guilt spiral. The fact is, NO ONE knows what it feels like to walk in my shoes or in the shoes of any caregiver. It's important to think before making a comment about a decision made by a caregiver. Believe me, every decision I make involving Mark is well-thought out, and tinged with a bit of guilt.

I don't think there is any possible way to live a guilt-free life as a caregiver. All we can do is take each day as it comes. Don't let our minds wander too far into the future. Build a team of resources to help, because you can't do it alone. And most importantly, offer yourself grace, you're doing the best you can.

CHAPTER 14

Walking By Faith

This has been the most difficult journey of my life, and I would not have survived it without my faith. There have been many times when I have felt completely distraught and have found myself on my knees praying to God to please lighten my load. I could physically feel the weight of what felt like the world on my shoulders. You know the saying, "God doesn't give you more than you can handle"? Well, at times, He did give me more than I could handle, and I yelled UNCLE.

The Bible verse that stayed with me throughout was Jeremiah 29:11, "For I know the plans I have for you. Plans to prosper you and not to harm you, plans to give you hope and a future."

I do believe that God loves me and even though this journey has been painful and even felt completely hopeless at times, I knew He was not trying to harm me. In total honesty, I did have moments when I questioned what the future could possibly look like. This is when I realized it's best to take things day by day. It quickly becomes overwhelming when you try to imagine the future.

Throughout this journey my faith has grown as I have seen miracles in Mark's recovery and we have been surrounded by family, friends, and even people we have never met who have held us in their prayers.

I believe if we look for them, there are signs sent to us by God. One day, while Mark was still residing in rehab, I was feeling extremely overwhelmed. Medical bills were pouring into my mailbox, I was questioning if I would even be able to care for Mark when the day arrived for him to come home, and worrying about my kids. I was a stressed out mess.

I made an appointment with my massage therapist, and dear friend Melissa at Lakeside Wellness and Apothecary. She suggested that I sit in the sauna before my massage. I connected my phone through Bluetooth and set my phone on Spotify to listen to music while I sweated it out in the sauna. Within five minutes of sitting in there, the Beatles' song, "Let it Be" came on. Mark's favorite band of all time is the Beatles. They're probably on my list of least favorites. My Spotify playlist didn't even have the Beatles listed, so I was a little irritated when this song started to play. My phone was outside of the sauna, so I had no choice, but to endure a Beatles song. However, as I listened to the words of this beautiful song, I started to cry. I knew this was a message being sent to me, and I needed to listen carefully to the lyrics.

Let it Be
By The Beatles
Written by Lennon and McCartney

When I find myself in times of trouble,
Mother Mary comes to me
Speaking words of wisdom, let it be.
And in my hour of darkness, she is
standing right in front of me
Speaking words of wisdom, let it be.
Let it be, let it be, let it be, let it be.
Whisper words of wisdom, let it be.

And when the broken-hearted people
living in the world agree
There will be an answer, let it be.
For though they may be parted, there is
still a chance that they will see
There will be an answer, let it be.

Let it be, let it be, let it be, let it be
There will be an answer, let it be.
Let it be, let it be, let it be, let it be
Whisper words of wisdom, let it be.

Let it be, let it be, let it be, let it be
Whisper words of wisdom, let it be.

And when the night is cloudy, there is
still a light that shines on me

Shine until tomorrow, let it be.
I wake up to the sound of music, Mother Mary comes to me
Speaking words of wisdom, let it be.

And let it be, let it be, let it be, yeah, let it be
There will be an answer, let it be.
Let it be, let it be, let it be, yeah, let it be
There will be an answer, let it be.

Let it be, let it be, let it be, let it be
Whisper words of wisdom, let it be.

Wow! This song spoke to me like no other.
Let it Be.

Those were the three words I needed to hear. I played this song over and over on repeat, as I let it soak in. I didn't need to worry about all of the what-if's, I needed to simply have faith, trust in God. And there would be an answer.

I don't have any tattoos, but I came very close to having the words "Let it Be" tattooed on my wrist! The irony is not lost on me that the message came to me from my least favorite band of all time. However, "Let it Be" is my favorite song now.

I've always believed that there are angels here on earth. One such angel made his presence known when I took Mark for a procedure to be done by a vascular surgeon. We knew that his left carotid was blocked, but didn't know if there might be a way to clear it or put in a stent.

On the day of his scheduled procedure, I was meeting Mark at the Heart Hospital, and he was being transported by van from the rehab. It was pouring rain as I drove to the hospital, and with each passing minute I was becoming more and more nervous about the procedure. I would be in the waiting room alone, and I had an overwhelming fear that the test would cause him to have another stroke. I think the chances of that happening were minimal, but there was no stopping this fear that had grabbed ahold of me.

The van was late, delayed by the terrible weather. Finally, they arrived and I watched this tiny man enter the hospital lobby pushing Mark in his wheelchair. This man may have been small in stature, but he had the biggest smile on his face that I've ever seen. He also had the most angelic glow about him. He told me that he was going to wait with me while Mark had his procedure done, and he did. There were a few other people in the waiting room with us, and this precious man kept us all entertained with stories and prayers. All of my fears melted away.

After what felt like only minutes, the medical staff came out to tell me that the procedure was finished and Mark had done well. Before he loaded Mark back into the van to return to the rehab, he asked if he could pray over us. Absolutely! He put his arms around both of us and said the most beautiful prayer. I don't remember the words he said, but I felt a peace come over me.

I believe God sent this angel to be there with me. Obviously, he was a human man, but there was something about him not like anyone I've ever met. I will never forget the kindness in his eyes, and the love he poured out on me and everyone else in that waiting room.

It's impossible to understand why God's plan was for Mark to suffer four strokes. I've learned that I can't question the "why," because I will never understand. I do know that through faith our family will get through this, and prosper in ways we never expected.

While I wish with all my heart that Mark was healthy and had never had a stroke, I see how this experience has changed all of us, and that much good has come from it. Past hurts from arguments have disappeared. Chris has matured and stepped up as an incredible caregiver and man of the house. Abby has been inspired to change her college major, and is now on track to becoming an Occupational Therapist. She wants to help people like Mark recover from injuries or illnesses.

Recently, a former neighbor passed away suddenly from a heart attack. Afterward, a friend commented to me that her husband said he'd rather die quickly like the former neighbor, rather than going through what Mark has gone through.

That has stayed in my thoughts. None of us get that choice of course, but after thinking about it, I am incredibly thankful that Mark survived, and I believe he is too. It's been a difficult journey and being realistic, it will always be a hard road, but this is the path God has given us and I know He has plans for us to prosper, and I am filled with hope for our future.

CHAPTER 15

Final Thoughts

As of this writing, Mark is 16 months post-stroke. He still goes to outpatient rehab five days a week, and continues to improve. He can now walk with a cane, and has some feeling returning to his right arm and hand. His speech is still difficult to understand, but he knows what he wants to tell us. It can be frustrating for him and for us, but we are finding ways to communicate.

The other day, he repeated the words "coffee and Danish" after me...and then kept saying them over and over. We both were so excited, I was dancing around as both of us chanted, "coffee, Danish, coffee, Danish!" Anyone looking in would've thought we had lost our minds. There is so much joy to be found even in the smallest of wins, and we will celebrate them all.

I've always loved music and how the lyrics of certain songs share what we feel in our hearts. I was in the car recently with Abby, when the song, "Stand by Me" came on. This is the song Mark and I danced to at our wedding, 34 years ago. Many artists have performed this beautiful song, but "our" rendition is by Mickey Gilley. It was the first song we danced to when we were newly dating. As I listened to the words, I thought to myself this song has always been the perfect song for us, today more than ever.

From the dark and uncertain days following Mark's strokes, to a future undoubtedly filled with many challenges, I am sure of one thing...*I will always stand by Mark.*

Stand By Me
Song by Ben E. King
Written by Ben E. King, Jerry Leiber, and Mike Stoller

When the night has come
And the land is dark
And the moon is the only light we'll see.
No, I won't be afraid
Oh, I won't be afraid
Just as long as you stand,
Stand By Me.

So darlin', darlin', stand by me
Oh, stand by me
Oh, stand
Stand by me, stand by me.
If the sky that we look upon
Should tumble and fall

Or the mountain should crumble to the sea
I won't cry, I won't cry
No, I won't shed a tear
Just as long as you stand
Stand By Me.

And darlin', darlin', stand by me
Oh, stand by me
Oh, stand now
Stand by me, stand by me
And darlin', darlin', stand by me
Oh, stand by me
Oh, stand now
Stand by me, stand by me.

Whenever you're in trouble won't you stand by me,
Oh, stand by me,
Won't you Stand By Me.

Made in the USA
Coppell, TX
18 July 2024

34758968R00083